Viruses: A Very Short Introduction

VERY SHORT INTRODUCTIONS are for anyone wanting a stimulating and accessible way in to a new subject. They are written by experts, and have been published in more than 25 languages worldwide.

The series began in 1995, and now represents a wide variety of topics in history, philosophy, religion, science, and the humanities. The VSI library now contains over 200 volumes—a Very Short Introduction to everything from ancient Egypt and Indian philosophy to conceptual art and cosmology—and will continue to grow to a library of around 300 titles.

Very Short Introductions available now:

ADVERTISING   Winston Fletcher
AFRICAN HISTORY
   John Parker and Richard Rathbone
AGNOSTICISM   Robin Le Poidevin
AMERICAN POLITICAL PARTIES
   AND ELECTIONS   L. Sandy Maisel
THE AMERICAN PRESIDENCY
   Charles O. Jones
ANARCHISM   Colin Ward
ANCIENT EGYPT   Ian Shaw
ANCIENT PHILOSOPHY
   Julia Annas
ANCIENT WARFARE
   Harry Sidebottom
ANGLICANISM   Mark Chapman
THE ANGLO-SAXON AGE
   John Blair
ANIMAL RIGHTS   David DeGrazia
ANTISEMITISM   Steven Beller
THE APOCRYPHAL GOSPELS
   Paul Foster
ARCHAEOLOGY   Paul Bahn
ARCHITECTURE   Andrew Ballantyne
ARISTOCRACY   William Doyle
ARISTOTLE   Jonathan Barnes
ART HISTORY   Dana Arnold
ART THEORY   Cynthia Freeland
ATHEISM   Julian Baggini
AUGUSTINE   Henry Chadwick
AUTISM   Uta Frith
BARTHES   Jonathan Culler
BEAUTY   Roger Scruton
BESTSELLERS   John Sutherland

THE BIBLE   John Riches
BIBLICAL ARCHAEOLOGY
   Eric H. Cline
BIOGRAPHY   Hermione Lee
THE BLUES   Elijah Wald
THE BOOK OF MORMON
   Terryl Givens
THE BRAIN   Michael O'Shea
BRITISH POLITICS   Anthony Wright
BUDDHA   Michael Carrithers
BUDDHISM   Damien Keown
BUDDHIST ETHICS   Damien Keown
CANCER   Nicholas James
CAPITALISM   James Fulcher
CATHOLICISM   Gerald O'Collins
THE CELTS   Barry Cunliffe
CHAOS   Leonard Smith
CHOICE THEORY
   Michael Allingham
CHRISTIAN ART   Beth Williamson
CHRISTIAN ETHICS   D. Stephen Long
CHRISTIANITY   Linda Woodhead
CITIZENSHIP   Richard Bellamy
CLASSICAL MYTHOLOGY
   Helen Morales
CLASSICS
   Mary Beard and John Henderson
CLAUSEWITZ   Michael Howard
THE COLD WAR   Robert McMahon
COMMUNISM   Leslie Holmes
CONSCIOUSNESS   Susan Blackmore
CONTEMPORARY ART
   Julian Stallabrass

CONTINENTAL PHILOSOPHY
    Simon Critchley
COSMOLOGY   Peter Coles
CRITICAL THEORY
    Stephen Bronner
THE CRUSADES
    Christopher Tyerman
CRYPTOGRAPHY
    Fred Piper and Sean Murphy
DADA AND SURREALISM
    David Hopkins
DARWIN   Jonathan Howard
THE DEAD SEA SCROLLS
    Timothy Lim
DEMOCRACY   Bernard Crick
DESCARTES   Tom Sorell
DESERTS   Nick Middleton
DESIGN   John Heskett
DINOSAURS   David Norman
DIPLOMACY   Joseph M. Siracusa
DOCUMENTARY FILM
    Patricia Aufderheide
DREAMING   J. Allan Hobson
DRUGS   Leslie Iversen
DRUIDS   Barry Cunliffe
EARLY MUSIC   Thomas Kelly
THE EARTH   Martin Redfern
ECONOMICS   Partha Dasgupta
EGYPTIAN MYTH   Geraldine Pinch
EIGHTEENTH-CENTURY BRITAIN
    Paul Langford
THE ELEMENTS   Philip Ball
EMOTION   Dylan Evans
EMPIRE   Stephen Howe
ENGELS   Terrell Carver
ENGLISH LITERATURE
    Jonathan Bate
EPIDEMIOLOGY   Roldolfo Saracci
ETHICS   Simon Blackburn
THE EUROPEAN UNION
    John Pinder and
    Simon Usherwood
EVOLUTION
    Brian and Deborah Charlesworth

EXISTENTIALISM   Thomas Flynn
FASCISM   Kevin Passmore
FASHION   Rebecca Arnold
FEMINISM   Margaret Walters
FILM MUSIC   Kathryn Kalinak
THE FIRST WORLD WAR
    Michael Howard
FOLK MUSIC   Mark Slobin
FORENSIC PSYCHOLOGY
    David Canter
FORENSIC SCIENCE   Jim Fraser
FOSSILS   Keith Thomson
FOUCAULT   Gary Gutting
FREE SPEECH   Nigel Warburton
FREE WILL   Thomas Pink
FRENCH LITERATURE
    John D. Lyons
THE FRENCH REVOLUTION
    William Doyle
FREUD   Anthony Storr
FUNDAMENTALISM   Malise Ruthven
GALAXIES   John Gribbin
GALILEO   Stillman Drake
GAME THEORY   Ken Binmore
GANDHI   Bhikhu Parekh
GENIUS   Andrew Robinson
GEOGRAPHY
    John Matthews and David Herbert
GEOPOLITICS   Klaus Dodds
GERMAN LITERATURE
    Nicholas Boyle
GERMAN PHILOSOPHY
    Andrew Bowie
GLOBAL CATASTROPHES
    Bill McGuire
GLOBAL WARMING   Mark Maslin
GLOBALIZATION   Manfred Steger
THE GREAT DEPRESSION AND
    THE NEW DEAL   Eric Rauchway
HABERMAS
    James Gordon Finlayson
HEGEL   Peter Singer
HEIDEGGER   Michael Inwood

HIEROGLYPHS Penelope Wilson
HINDUISM Kim Knott
HISTORY John H. Arnold
THE HISTORY OF ASTRONOMY
    Michael Hoskin
THE HISTORY OF LIFE
    Michael Benton
THE HISTORY OF MEDICINE
    William Bynum
THE HISTORY OF TIME
    Leofranc Holford-Strevens
HIV/AIDS Alan Whiteside
HOBBES Richard Tuck
HUMAN EVOLUTION
    Bernard Wood
HUMAN RIGHTS Andrew Clapham
HUMANISM Stephen Law
HUME A. J. Ayer
IDEOLOGY Michael Freeden
INDIAN PHILOSOPHY
    Sue Hamilton
INFORMATION Luciano Floridi
INNOVATION
    Mark Dodgson and David Gann
INTELLIGENCE Ian J. Deary
INTERNATIONAL MIGRATION
    Khalid Koser
INTERNATIONAL RELATIONS
    Paul Wilkinson
ISLAM Malise Ruthven
ISLAMIC HISTORY Adam Silverstein
JOURNALISM Ian Hargreaves
JUDAISM Norman Solomon
JUNG Anthony Stevens
KABBALAH Joseph Dan
KAFKA Ritchie Robertson
KANT Roger Scruton
KEYNES Robert Skidelsky
KIERKEGAARD Patrick Gardiner
THE KORAN Michael Cook
LANDSCAPES AND
    GEOMORPHOLOGY
    Andrew Goudie and Heather Viles
LATE ANTIQUITY Gillian Clark
LAW Raymond Wacks

THE LAWS OF THERMODYNAMICS
    Peter Atkins
LEADERSHIP Keith Grint
LINCOLN Allen C. Guelzo
LINGUISTICS Peter Matthews
LITERARY THEORY Jonathan Culler
LOCKE John Dunn
LOGIC Graham Priest
MACHIAVELLI Quentin Skinner
THE MARQUIS DE SADE
    John Phillips
MARTIN LUTHER Scott H. Hendrix
MARX Peter Singer
MATHEMATICS Timothy Gowers
THE MEANING OF LIFE
    Terry Eagleton
MEDICAL ETHICS Tony Hope
MEDIEVAL BRITAIN
    John Gillingham and
    Ralph A. Griffiths
MEMORY Jonathan K. Foster
MICHAEL FARADAY
    Frank A. J. L. James
MODERN ART David Cottington
MODERN CHINA Rana Mitter
MODERN IRELAND Senia Pašeta
MODERN JAPAN
    Christopher Goto-Jones
MODERNISM
    Christopher Butler
MOLECULES Philip Ball
MORMONISM
    Richard Lyman Bushman
MUHAMMAD Jonathan A. C. Brown
MUSIC Nicholas Cook
MYTH Robert A. Segal
NATIONALISM Steven Grosby
NELSON MANDELA Elleke Boehmer
NEOLIBERALISM
    Manfred Steger and Ravi Roy
THE NEW TESTAMENT
    Luke Timothy Johnson
THE NEW TESTAMENT AS
    LITERATURE Kyle Keefer
NEWTON Robert Iliffe

NIETZSCHE Michael Tanner

NINETEENTH-CENTURY BRITAIN
Christopher Harvie and
H. C. G. Matthew

THE NORMAN CONQUEST
George Garnett

NORTH AMERICAN INDIANS
Theda Perdue and Michael D. Green

NORTHERN IRELAND
Marc Mulholland

NOTHING Frank Close

NUCLEAR POWER Maxwell Irvine

NUCLEAR WEAPONS
Joseph M. Siracusa

NUMBERS Peter M. Higgins

THE OLD TESTAMENT
Michael D. Coogan

ORGANIZATIONS Mary Jo Hatch

PAGANISM Owen Davies

PARTICLE PHYSICS Frank Close

PAUL E. P. Sanders

PENTECOSTALISM William K. Kay

PHILOSOPHY Edward Craig

PHILOSOPHY OF LAW
Raymond Wacks

PHILOSOPHY OF SCIENCE
Samir Okasha

PHOTOGRAPHY Steve Edwards

PLANETS David A. Rothery

PLATO Julia Annas

POLITICAL PHILOSOPHY
David Miller

POLITICS Kenneth Minogue

POSTCOLONIALISM Robert Young

POSTMODERNISM Christopher Butler

POSTSTRUCTURALISM
Catherine Belsey

PREHISTORY Chris Gosden

PRESOCRATIC PHILOSOPHY
Catherine Osborne

PRIVACY Raymond Wacks

PROGRESSIVISM Walter Nugent

PSYCHIATRY Tom Burns

PSYCHOLOGY
Gillian Butler and Freda McManus

PURITANISM Francis J. Bremer

THE QUAKERS Pink Dandelion

QUANTUM THEORY
John Polkinghorne

RACISM Ali Rattansi

THE REAGAN REVOLUTION Gil Troy

THE REFORMATION Peter Marshall

RELATIVITY Russell Stannard

RELIGION IN AMERICA Timothy Beal

THE RENAISSANCE Jerry Brotton

RENAISSANCE ART
Geraldine A. Johnson

ROMAN BRITAIN Peter Salway

THE ROMAN EMPIRE
Christopher Kelly

ROMANTICISM Michael Ferber

ROUSSEAU Robert Wokler

RUSSELL A. C. Grayling

RUSSIAN LITERATURE Catriona Kelly

THE RUSSIAN REVOLUTION
S. A. Smith

SCHIZOPHRENIA
Chris Frith and Eve Johnstone

SCHOPENHAUER
Christopher Janaway

SCIENCE AND RELIGION
Thomas Dixon

THE SCIENTIFIC REVOLUTION
Lawrence M. Principe

SCOTLAND Rab Houston

SEXUALITY Véronique Mottier

SHAKESPEARE Germaine Greer

SIKHISM Eleanor Nesbitt

SOCIAL AND CULTURAL
ANTHROPOLOGY
John Monaghan and Peter Just

SOCIALISM Michael Newman

SOCIOLOGY Steve Bruce

SOCRATES C. C. W. Taylor

THE SOVIET UNION
Stephen Lovell

THE SPANISH CIVIL WAR
Helen Graham

SPANISH LITERATURE Jo Labanyi

SPINOZA   Roger Scruton
STATISTICS   David J. Hand
STUART BRITAIN   John Morrill
SUPERCONDUCTIVITY
    Stephen Blundell
TERRORISM
    Charles Townshend
THEOLOGY   David F. Ford
THOMAS AQUINAS   Fergus Kerr
TOCQUEVILLE
    Harvey C. Mansfield
TRAGEDY   Adrian Poole
THE TUDORS   John Guy
TWENTIETH-CENTURY BRITAIN
    Kenneth O. Morgan

THE UNITED NATIONS
    Jussi M. Hanhimäki
THE U.S. CONGRESS
    Donald A. Ritchie
UTOPIANISM
    Lyman Tower Sargent
THE VIKINGS   Julian Richards
VIRUSES   Dorothy H. Crawford
WITCHCRAFT   Malcolm Gaskill
WITTGENSTEIN   A. C. Grayling
WORLD MUSIC   Philip Bohlman
THE WORLD TRADE ORGANIZATION
    Amrita Narlikar
WRITING AND SCRIPT
    Andrew Robinson

Available soon:

DICTIONARIES   Lynda Mugglestone
DEVELOPMENTAL BIOLOGY
    Lewis Wolpert
PROTESTANTISM   Mark A. Noll

DERRIDA   Simon Glendinning
MADNESS   Andrew Scull
MULTICULTURALISM   Ali Rattansi

For more information visit our website

www.oup.com/vsi/

Dorothy H. Crawford

VIRUSES

A Very Short Introduction

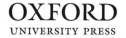
OXFORD
UNIVERSITY PRESS

OXFORD
UNIVERSITY PRESS

Great Clarendon Street, Oxford ox2 6DP

Oxford University Press is a department of the University of Oxford.
It furthers the University's objective of excellence in research, scholarship, and
education by publishing worldwide in

Oxford New York

Auckland Cape Town Dar es Salaam Hong Kong Karachi
Kuala Lumpur Madrid Melbourne Mexico City Nairobi
New Delhi Shanghai Taipei Toronto

With offices in

Argentina Austria Brazil Chile Czech Republic France Greece
Guatemala Hungary Italy Japan Poland Portugal Singapore
South Korea Switzerland Thailand Turkey Ukraine Vietnam

Oxford is a registered trade mark of Oxford University Press
in the UK and in certain other countries

Published in the United States
by Oxford University Press Inc., New York

British Library Cataloguing in Publication Data

Data available

Library of Congress Cataloging in Publication Data

Data available

Typeset by SPI Publisher Services, Pondicherry, India
Printed in Great Britain by
Ashford Colour Press Ltd, Gosport, Hampshire

ISBN 978-0-19-957485-8

1 3 5 7 9 10 8 6 4 2

Contents

Acknowledgements   xi

List of illustrations   xiii

Introduction   xv

1   What are viruses?   1

2   Viruses are everywhere   16

3   Kill or be killed   25

4   Emerging virus infections   34

5   Epidemics and pandemics   51

6   Persistent viruses   65

7   Tumour viruses   83

8   Turning the tables   102

9   Viruses past, present, and future   119

Glossary   133

Further reading   147

Index   151

Acknowledgements

I would like to thank the following for professional advice: Dr Tanzina Haque, Dr Ingo Johannessen, and Professor Peter Simmonds for their expert advice on viruses; and Jeanne Bell, Frances Fowler, Karen McAualy, and Alero Thomas for their valuable comments on the manuscript. I am also indebted to Latha Menon and Emma Marchant at Oxford University Press for their help with the production of this book.

List of illustrations

1   The structure of viruses **5**
From D. Greenwood et al. (eds.),
Medical Microbiology, 16th edn.
(Churchill Livingstone, 2002), p. 23,
fig. 2.16
© Elsevier

2   The comparative sizes of a
typical bacterium and
representative viruses **6**
From L. Collier and J. S. Oxford
Human Virology (OUP, 1993), p. 4,
fig. 1.1
© Oxford University Press

3   The structure of DNA **7**
From B. and D. Charlesworth,
*Evolution: A Very Short
Introduction* (OUP, 2003), p. 25,
fig. 5b
© Oxford University Press

4   The retrovirus infectious
cycle **10**
© www.clontech.com

5   Biogeochemical cycling
showing the viral shunt **20**
From *Nature* 437 (2005),
fig. 3. Adapted by
permission from Macmillan
Publishers Ltd.

6   The cholera cycle **23**
From D. H. Crawford, *Deadly
Companions* (OUP, 2007), p. 136,
fig. 5.3
© Oxford University Press

7   Portals of virus entry into the
human body **26**

8   The cumulative number of
emerging virus infections in
humans, 1988 to 2007 **35**
From Zuckerman et al. (eds.),
*Principles and Practice of Clinical
Virology*, 6th edn. (Wiley and
Blackwell, 2009), p. 70, fig. 4.2
© John Wiley & Sons Ltd.

9   The emergence of SARS in
Hong Kong, February to June
2003 **36**
From *SARS in Hong Kong: From
Experience to Action*, Report of the
SARS Expert Committee Chapter 3
(October 2003). SARS Expert
Committee

10 The estimated number of
AIDS-related deaths
worldwide, 1980 to 2000 **36**
Source: UNAIDS

11 The worldwide distribution of dengue fever, 2010 **46**
© WHO 2010. All rights reserved

12 Croup hospitalizations in children under 15 in the USA, 1981–2002 **58**
From C. S. D. Roxborgh et al, 'Trends in pneumonia and empysema in Scottish children in the past 25 years', *BMJ* Vol. 93 (April 1, 2008.) with permission from BMJ publishing Group Ltd

13 CD4 count and viral load during acute, asymptomatic, and symptomatic phases of HIV infection **75**
From A. Mindel and M. Tenant-Flowers, 'Natural History and Management of early HIV infection', *ABC of Aids* (2001), with permission from BMJ Publishing Group Ltd.

14 World map showing the prevalence of HBV and HCV infections **79**
Cancer Research UK, http://info.cancer-research.org/cancerstats. Source: WHO

15 World map showing the prevalence of HTLV-1 infection **89**
Cancer Research UK, http://info.cancer-research.org/cancerstats.

16 Burkitt's map of the distribution of Burkitt's lymphoma in Africa **92**
From D. Burkitt, 'Determining the Climatic Limitations of Children's Cancer Common in Africa', *British Medical Journal*, 2 (1962): 1019–23, with permission from BMJ Publishing Group

17 Age-standardized incidence and mortality for cervical cancer by world region, 2002 **100**
Cancer Research UK, http://info.cancer-research.org/cancerstats. Source: GLOBOCAN

18 'The Cow-Pock-or-The Wonderful Effects of the New Inoculation', by James Gillray, 1802 **105**
Courtesy of the Library of Congress

19 The yellow fever transmission cycle **123**
From D. H. Crawford, *The Invisible Enemy* (OUP, 2000), p. 26, fig. 1.4
© Oxford University Press

Introduction

This book is an introduction to viruses written for the general reader. The first two chapters introduce viruses, their structure and diversity, as well as where and how they live and their effects, from those on the infected individual to the whole planet. The book then outlines the constant battle between viruses and the immune system of the infected individual, followed by a series of chapters about infection by specific groups of viruses, be they emerging, epidemic, or pandemic viruses or those that persist in the body for a lifetime, some of which may cause tumours. Later chapters look at how our knowledge of viruses has advanced through the ages and how the recent molecular revolution has enhanced our ability to isolate new viruses and to diagnose and treat virus infections. The final chapter takes a historical perspective on the changing pattern of virus infections through the ages and speculates about how humans and viruses might interact in the future.

As far as possible, the author has avoided the use of specialist and technical terms in the text, but where these are unavoidable their meaning is explained in the glossary. This also includes the derivation of virus names. In addition, a list of suggestions for further reading is included at the end of the book.

Chapter 1
What are viruses?

> The microbe is so very small
> You cannot make him out at all,
> But many sanguine people hope
> To see him through a microscope.
> His jointed tongue that lies beneath
> A hundred curious rows of teeth;
> His seven tufted tails with lots
> Of lovely pink and purple spots,
> On each of which a pattern stands,
> Composed of forty separate bands;
> His eyebrows of a tender green;
> All these have never yet been seen –
> But Scientists, who ought to know,
> Assure us that they must be so...
> Oh! let us never, never doubt
> What nobody is sure about.
>
> 'The Microbe' (1896), Hilaire Belloc

Primitive microbes evolved on Earth approximately three billion years ago but were isolated by humans only in the late 19th century, around 20 years before Hilaire Belloc wrote 'The Microbe'. Written to amuse, the poem nonetheless reflects the scepticism of the times. It must have taken a huge leap of faith for people to accept that tiny, living organisms were responsible for diseases that had hitherto been attributed variously to the will of the gods, the alignment of planets, or miasmic vapours emanating from swamps and decomposing organic material. Of course, this realization did not dawn overnight, but as more and more bacteria were identified, the 'germ theory' took hold, and by the beginning of the 20th century it was widely accepted even in non-scientific circles that microbes could cause disease.

Key to this momentous leap in understanding were technical developments in microscopes made by the Dutch lens-maker Antonie van Leeuwenhoek (1632–1723) in the 16th century. He was the first to visualize microbes, but it was not until the mid-1800s that Louis Pasteur (1822–95) working in Paris and Robert Koch (1843–1910) in Berlin carried out the ground-breaking scientific work which established 'germs' as the cause of infectious diseases, earning them the title 'the founding fathers of microbiology'. Pasteur was instrumental in dispelling the general belief in 'spontaneous generation', that is, the generation of life from inorganic material. At the time, the growth of moulds on stored food and drink was a particular problem. Pasteur demonstrated that this could be prevented in broth first by boiling and then by placing it in a chamber with filters to exclude the entry of any particulate material from the air. This demonstrated the existence of airborne microscopic 'germs'. In 1876, Koch isolated the first bacterium, *Bacillus anthracis*, and soon developed methods for growing microbes in the laboratory.

One after another, feared diseases like anthrax, tuberculosis, cholera, diphtheria, tetanus, and syphilis delivered up their secrets as their causative microbes were identified and characterized. It became clear that bacteria have a structure similar to mammalian cells, most having a cell wall surrounding cytoplasm that contains a single, coiled, circular molecule of DNA. The majority of bacteria are free living, meaning that they can manufacture all the proteins they need, metabolize, and divide without the help of other organisms.

Despite this success in isolating pathogenic bacteria, there remained a group of infectious diseases which stubbornly resisted all attempts to isolate their causative organisms, including common and lethal infections such as smallpox, measles, mumps, rubella, and flu. These microbes were obviously very small as they passed through filters that trapped bacteria, and in consequence were called 'filterable agents'. At the time, most scientists thought these were just tiny bacteria.

In 1876, Adolf Mayer (1843–1942), director of the Agricultural Experimental Station in Wageningen, Holland, began to investigate a new disease of tobacco plants which was devastating the valuable Dutch tobacco industry. He called it 'tobacco mosaic disease' because of the mottled pattern it produces on the diseased plant's leaves. Mayer was the first to show that the disease was infectious when he transmitted it to a healthy plant by rubbing its leaves with sap extracted from a diseased plant. He concluded that the disease was caused by a very small bacterium or a toxin, but he did not pursue the research any further.

Later, biologist Dmitry Ivanovsky (1864–1920) also worked on tobacco mosaic disease at the University of St Petersburg in Russia. He called the disease 'wildfire', and in 1892 demonstrated that its causative agent passed through filters that trapped bacteria and, like Mayer, suggested it was caused by a chemical toxin produced by a bacterium.

Then in 1898, Martinus Beijerinck (1851–1931), a microbiology teacher at the Agricultural School in Wageningen, followed up on Mayer's experiments. Unaware of Ivanovsky's work, he repeated the filter experiments that demonstrated a tiny filterable agent, but he further showed that the agent grew in dividing cells and regained its full strength each time it infected a plant. He concluded that it must be a living microbe, and was the first to coin the name *virus*, from the Latin meaning a poison, venom, or slimy fluid.

By the beginning of the 20th century, viruses were defined as a group of microbes that were infectious, filterable, and required living cells for their propagation, but the nature of their structure remained a mystery. In the 1930s, tobacco mosaic virus was obtained in crystalline form, suggesting that viruses were purely composed of protein, but shortly afterwards a nucleic acid component was discovered and shown to be essential for infectivity. However, it was not until the invention of the electron microscope in 1939 that viruses were first visualized and their structure elucidated, showing them to be a unique class of microbes.

Viruses are not cells but particles. They consist of a protein coat which surrounds and protects their genetic material, or, as the famous immunologist Sir Peter Medawar (1915–87) termed it, 'a piece of bad news wrapped up in protein'. The whole structure is called a *virion* and the outer coat is called the *capsid*. Capsids come in various shapes and sizes, each characteristic of the virus family to which it belongs. They are built up of protein subunits called *capsomeres* and it is the arrangement of these around the central genetic material that determines the shape of the virion. For example, poxviruses are brick-shaped, herpesviruses are icosahedral (twenty-sided spheres), the rabies virus is bullet-shaped, and tobacco mosaic virus is long and thin like a rod (Figure 1). Some viruses have an outer layer surrounding the capsid called an *envelope*.

Most viruses are too small to be seen under a light microscope. In general, they are around 100 to 500 times smaller than bacteria, varying in size from 20 to 300 nanometres in diameter (nm; 1 nm is a thousand millionth of a metre) (Figure 2). However, the recently discovered giant, the mimivirus (short for 'microbe-mimicking virus'; of which more later), is an exception, with a diameter of around 700 nm; larger than some bacteria.

Inside the virus capsid is its genetic material, or *genome*, which is either RNA or DNA depending on the type of virus (Figure 3). The

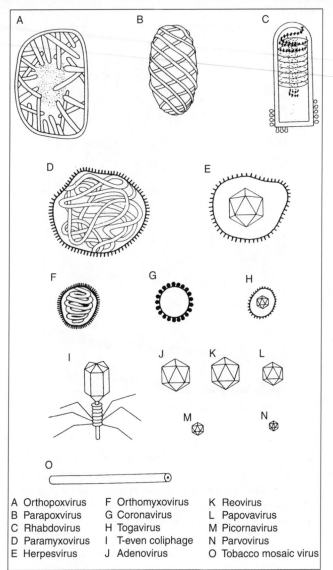

A Orthopoxvirus
B Parapoxvirus
C Rhabdovirus
D Paramyxovirus
E Herpesvirus
F Orthomyxovirus
G Coronavirus
H Togavirus
I T-even coliphage
J Adenovirus
K Reovirus
L Papovavirus
M Picornavirus
N Parvovirus
O Tobacco mosaic virus

1. **The structure of viruses**

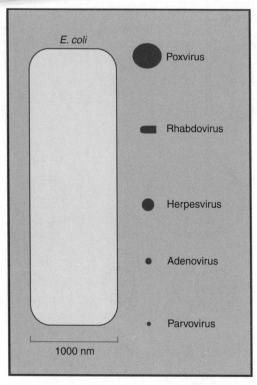

2. The comparative sizes of a typical bacterium and representative viruses

genome contains the virus's genes, which carry the code for making new viruses, and transmits these inherited characteristics to the next generation. Viruses usually have between 2 and 200 genes, but again mimivirus is most unusual in having an estimated 600 to 1,000 genes, even more than many bacteria.

Cells of free-living organisms, including bacteria, contain a variety of organelles essential for life such as ribosomes that manufacture proteins, mitochondria or other structures that generate energy,

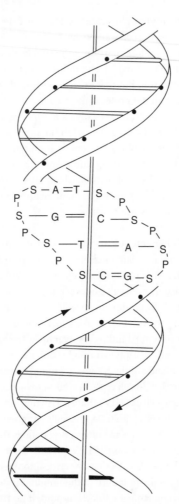

3. The structure of DNA, showing the two complementary strands that form the helix. The backbone of each strand is composed of molecules of the sugar deoxyribose (S) that are linked to each other through phosphate molecules (P). Each sugar is connected to a nucleotide molecule, and these form the 'letters' of the genetic alphabet. These are: adenine (A), guanine (G), cytosine (C), and thymine (T)

and complex membranes for transporting molecules within the cell, and also across the cell wall. Viruses, not being cells, have none of these and are therefore inert until they infect a living cell. Virus particles resemble seeds which can only spring into life when they find the right soil. But unlike seeds, viruses do not carry the genes to code for all the proteins they require to 'germinate' and complete their life cycle. So they hijack a cell's organelles and use what they need, often killing the cell in the process. This lifestyle means that viruses are obliged to obtain essential components of their life cycle from other living things and are therefore called *obligate parasites*. Even mimivirus, which infects amoebae, has to borrow the amoeba's organelles to manufacture its proteins in order to assemble new mimiviruses.

Plant viruses either enter cells through a break in the cell wall or are injected by a sap-sucking insect vector like an aphid. They then spread very efficiently from cell to cell via plasmodesmata, the pores that transport molecules between cells. In contrast, animal viruses infect cells by binding to specific receptor molecules on the cell surface. The cell receptor is like a lock, and only viruses that carry the right receptor-binding key can open the lock and enter that particular cell. Receptor molecules differ from one type of virus to another, and although some are found on most cells, others are restricted to certain cell types. A well-known example is human immunodeficiency virus (HIV) that carries the entry key for the CD4 lock, so only cells with CD4 molecules on their surface can be infected by HIV. This specific interaction defines the outcome of the infection, and in the case of HIV leads to destruction of CD4-positive 'helper' T cells that are critical to the immune response. This results in failure of the immune system, with the risk of serious opportunistic infections and, if no treatment is given, eventual death of the individual.

Once a virus has bound to its cellular receptor, the capsid penetrates the cell and its genome (DNA or RNA) is released into the cell cytoplasm. The main 'aim' of a virus is to reproduce successfully, and to do this its genetic material must download the information it carries. Mostly, this will take place in the cell's nucleus where the virus can access the molecules it needs to begin manufacturing its own proteins. However, some large viruses, like pox viruses, carry genes for the enzymes they need to make their proteins and so are more self-sufficient and can complete the whole life cycle in the cytoplasm.

Once inside a cell, DNA viruses simply masquerade as pieces of cellular DNA, and their genes are transcribed and translated using as much of the cell's machinery as they require for their own virus production line. The viral DNA code is transcribed into RNA messages which are read and translated into individual viral proteins by the cell's ribosomes. The separate virus components are then assembled into thousands of new viruses which are often so tightly packed inside the cell that it eventually bursts open and releases them, inevitably killing the cell. Alternatively, new viruses leave rather more sedately by budding through the cell membrane. In the latter case, the cell may survive and act as a reservoir of infection.

RNA viruses are one step ahead of DNA viruses in already having their genetic code as RNA. As they carry enzymes that enable their RNA to be copied and translated into proteins, they are not so dependent on cellular enzymes and can often complete their life cycle in the cytoplasm without causing major disruption to the cell.

Retroviruses are a family of RNA viruses that include HIV and have evolved a unique trick for establishing a lifelong infection of a cell while hiding from immune attack. Retrovirus particles contain an enzyme called *reverse transcriptase* which, once inside a cell, converts their RNA to DNA (Figure 4). This viral DNA can then join, or *integrate*, into the cell's DNA using another enzyme carried by the virus called *integrase*. The integrated viral sequence is called the *provirus*, and is effectively archived in the cell, remaining there permanently to be copied along with cellular DNA when the cell

Retrovirus lifecycle

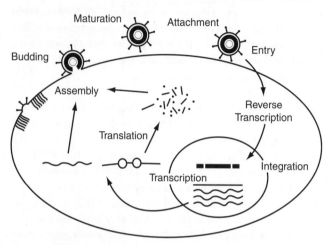

4. The retrovirus infectious cycle, showing viral entry into a cell followed by reverse transcription, integration, transcription and translation of the genome, virus assembly, and budding of new particles from the cell surface

divides. The provirus is inherited by the two daughter cells, so building up a store of infected cells inside its host. At any time, a provirus can manufacture new viruses which bud from the cell surface, but in this instance it kills the cell.

In mammalian cells, the process of copying DNA during cell division is highly regulated, with a proof-reading system and several checkpoints in place to detect damaged or miscopied DNA and to correct the mistakes. If the damage is too great to be corrected, cells have an 'auto-destruct' programme called *apoptosis* that induces death rather than allowing the cell to pass on its faulty DNA. Despite these checks, mistakes slip through, causing mutations to be replicated and passed on to future generations (see Box 1).

Box 1

Molecular evolution

Virus genes accumulate mutations over time

```
A ..GAAGCACTCTACCTCGTGTGCGGGGATCGAGGCTTATTCTACACACCCAAGC...
      X        X            X          X                    X
B ..GAAGCTCTCTACCTAGTGTGCGGGGAACGAGGCTTCTTCTACACACCCAAGA...
    X  X      X            X          X  X  X              X
C ..GAGGCGCTGTACCTGGTGTGCGGGGAGCGCGGCTTTTTTTATACACCCAAGT...
```

A vs B: 5 mutations across 50 sites = 10% difference
B vs C: 10 mutations across 50 sites = 20% difference

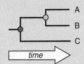

An example of evolution of a viral gene over time. This
information is used to construct an evolutionary tree in which the
length of the lines denotes the time since the last common
ancestor. (Kindly provided by Professor Paul Sharp, University of
Edinburgh)

What are viruses?

In humans, mutations arise at a rate of one in every million
nucleotides (called base pairs, of which our DNA has 3×10^9) per
generation, but they appear more frequently in viruses. This is
partly because, compared to the human generation time of around
30 years, viruses can reproduce in a day or two. Also, there is no
proof-reading system for RNA, so viruses with an RNA genome
have a high mutation rate of around one in every thousand base
pairs per generation. Thus, every time a virus infects a cell, its DNA
or RNA may be copied thousands of times, and as each new strand
is incorporated into a new virus particle, every round of infection
throws up several mutant viruses. This high mutation rate in
viruses is their lifeline; in some, it is essential for their survival.
Each round of infection produces some viruses that are non-viable
due to mutations that interrupt the function of essential genes, and

others with mutations that cause no change in function. However, a few of the offspring will have beneficial mutations, giving them a selective advantage over their siblings. The benefit may result in any number of advantages, including a heightened ability to fight, or hide from, immune attack; to survive and spread between hosts; to resist antiviral drugs; or to reproduce at a faster rate. Whatever the advantage, it will lead to that particular mutant virus outstripping its siblings and eventually taking over in the population. Examples of this are common, particularly among RNA viruses like measles, which has been infecting the human population for around 2,000 years. Despite this, scientists calculate that the present-day measles strain arose only about 100 to 200 years ago. Presumably, this virus was 'fitter' than its predecessor in some way; perhaps it had better spreading powers, and so eventually replaced the former strain worldwide. Another famous example is HIV, which rapidly evolves resistance to the drugs used to control the infection. In practice, this means that several antiretroviral drugs have to be used together for effective treatment, and even then drug resistance is a growing problem. When a drug-resistant virus is transmitted to an uninfected person, the new infection is much more difficult to control. The same process has also foiled all attempts to make an effective HIV vaccine.

Analysing the mutations in its genome is a useful way of tracking a virus's history. The molecular clock hypothesis, which was developed in the 1960s, states that the mutation rate per generation is constant for any given gene. In other words, as applied to viruses, two samples of the same type of virus isolated at the same time from different sources will have evolved for the same length of time since their common ancestor. Since they will both have been accumulating mutations at a constant rate, the degree of difference between their gene sequences provides a measure of the time that has passed since their common ancestor. This way of measuring evolutionary time has been verified in higher life forms by comparing the dates of origin estimated by the molecular clock with those estimated from fossil records, but unfortunately viruses leave no such records. Nevertheless, scientists use the molecular clock to estimate the time of origin of certain viruses, and plot evolutionary (or phylogenetic) trees showing their degree of relatedness to other viruses. Because viruses have a high mutation rate, significant evolutionary change, estimated at around 1% per year for HIV, can be measured over a short timescale. Since the rate of change for any particular gene is fairly constant, the longer the gene has been evolving, the more mutations it will acquire. So the history of two related viruses can be traced in time back to their common ancestor using this so-called 'molecular clock'. The technique was used to uncover the history of the measles virus. It was also used to discover that smallpox virus is most closely related to the pox viruses of camels and gerbils, suggesting that all three arose from a common ancestor around 5,000 to 10,000 years ago.

Because virus particles are inert, without the ability to generate energy or manufacture proteins independently, they are not generally regarded as living organisms. Nonetheless, they are pieces of genetic material that parasitize cells, very efficiently exploiting the cells' internal machinery to reproduce themselves. So how and when did these cellular hijackers originate?

This is a controversy to which we do not yet know the answer, although it is now generally accepted that viruses are truly ancient. The fact that viruses sharing common features infect organisms in all three domains of life – Archaea, Bacteria, and Eukarya – suggests that they evolved before these domains separated from their common ancestor, called the 'last universal cellular ancestor' (LUCA). There are three main theories to explain the origin of viruses.

The first theory suggests that viruses were the first organisms to arise in the 'primordial soup' around four billion years ago. Given that modern-day viruses are obligate parasites that must infect a cell and use its organelles in order to reproduce, this theory proposes that large DNA viruses, for example poxviruses, may represent a previously free-living life form that has now lost its ability to reproduce independently.

The second and third theories both propose that viruses originated before the advent of DNA, when primitive, pre-LUCA cells used RNA as their genetic material. One theory suggests that viruses derived from escaped fragments of this RNA that acquired a protein coat and became infectious. The other theory proposes that viruses represent primitive RNA cells that have been reduced to a parasitic lifestyle through being out-competed when other, more complex cells evolved. Both these theories are easier to believe when considering RNA rather than DNA viruses, and so scientists have proposed that DNA viruses evolved from their more ancient RNA counterparts. This suggestion is supported by the existence of retroviruses, with their ability to transcribe RNA into DNA. In so doing, they reverse the more usual flow of genetic information that goes from DNA to RNA to protein. No one believed this was possible until the retrovirus reverse transcriptase enzyme was discovered in 1970. Perhaps retroviruses represent the missing link between the ancient RNA and modern DNA worlds. Virus evolution is a fascinating field of research which remains a hot topic, but until it is resolved, the question of how viruses fit into the tree of life remains unanswered.

During the early 20th century, criteria were developed for determining whether an infectious agent was in fact a virus. The agent had to pass through filters that retained bacteria, had to be infectious, and unable to grow in cultures that supported bacterial growth. Virus identification was greatly enhanced by the invention of the electron microscope in the late 1930s, and this was thereafter routinely used to discover new viruses and characterize their sizes and shapes more precisely. Once it was appreciated that viruses carried either DNA or RNA, but never both, a system of classification was devised based on the following criteria to assign viruses into families, genera, and species:

- the type of nucleic acid (DNA or RNA);
- the shape of the virus capsid;
- the capsid diameter and/or number of capsomeres;
- the presence or absence of an envelope.

Since the early 1980s, when the first virus genome was fully sequenced, this has become a routine technique that provides valuable information for virus classification. Indeed, with increasingly sophisticated methods for virus discovery, many viruses are now identified long before their actual physical structure is visualized. In these cases, the molecular structure of the DNA or RNA is compared with that of other known viruses to assign the new virus to a family.

The discovery of the hepatitis C virus in 1989 was the first that used molecular probes. After the isolation of hepatitis A and B viruses, people with symptoms characteristic of viral hepatitis regularly presented at the clinic but were not infected with either of these viruses. This disease was called non-A, non-B hepatitis, inevitably leading scientists to predict the existence of another hepatitis virus. They were determined to find this elusive virus, so they cloned segments of RNA directly from the blood of a chimpanzee that had been experimentally infected with material from a patient with non-A, non-B hepatitis. They found a series of unique RNA sequences which together gave a genome length, composition, and organization typical of the flavivirus family, yet distinct from any others known at the time. This 'new' virus was called hepatitis C virus.

With these new techniques for identifying viruses, virus discovery has gone way beyond the search for the causes of disease to encompass the wider environment where we find viruses in abundance. The next chapter will explore the extent and complexity of this 'virosphere' in which we live.

Chapter 2
Viruses are everywhere

Until a short while ago, most virus discovery programmes were fuelled by attempts to find the causative agents of human, animal, and plant diseases, well-known recent examples being SARS (severe acute respiratory syndrome) and AIDS (acquired immune deficiency syndrome). This has given the impression that viruses generally cause disease, but molecular techniques for large-scale environmental genome sampling show that this is far from true. It is now clear that viruses form a huge biomass of enormous variety and complexity in the environment, the whole being aptly termed the 'virosphere'.

Microbes are by far the most abundant life form on Earth. Globally, there are about 5×10^{30} bacteria, and viruses are at least 10 times more common – thus making viruses the most numerous microbes on Earth. In other words, there are more viruses in the world than all other forms of life added together. Viruses are also staggeringly diverse, with an estimated 100 million different types. Perhaps it is not surprising, then, to find that they have invaded every niche occupied by living things, including the most inhospitable places, such as hydrothermal vents in the deep oceans, under the polar ice caps, and in salt marshes and acid lakes. These are all locations favoured by certain archaean species known as 'extremophiles'. The viruses that infect archaea and bacteria are called bacteriophages (or phages for short) and have a

certain structural resemblance to a rocket on a launch pad
(see Chapter 1, Figure 1).

Recent virus hunting has uncovered viruses of astonishingly varied
shapes and sizes, and one of the most remarkable is the mimivirus,
introduced in Chapter 1. During an investigation of a pneumonia
outbreak in 1992, this virus was found by chance inside amoebae
living in a water-cooling tower in Bradford, UK. This giant virus
was at first assumed to be a bacterium living inside the amoeba cell.
As such, it seemed of little interest and was set aside, until several
years later when scientists sequenced its genome and revealed the
largest virus ever known. Among its approximately 600 genes, of
which 75% are of completely unknown origin and function, there
are genes involved in genome translation never found in viruses
before. Only a handful of the mimivirus genes have known relatives
among those of bacteria, archaea, and eukaryotes, but these few
have been used to map its position in the tree of life. Surprisingly,
mimivirus genes are most similar to those of eukaryotes so that this
virus falls into an evolutionary position at a point before the animal
and plant kingdoms split, and therefore clearly has a very long and
interesting history (see Box 2).

The discovery of mimivirus was not just a freak event. We now
know that natural, untreated water is teeming with viruses and, in
fact, viruses are the most abundant life forms in the oceans. The
oceans cover 65% of the globe's surface and, as there are up to
10 billion viruses per one litre of sea water, the whole ocean
contains around 4×10^{30} – enough, when laid side by side, to
span 10 million light years.

So what is this mêlée of viruses doing in the oceans, and is it of
any importance?

The study of microbial oceanography is still in its infancy but, by
using robots to collect series of samples through time and water
depths, and large-scale genomic analysis, we are beginning to

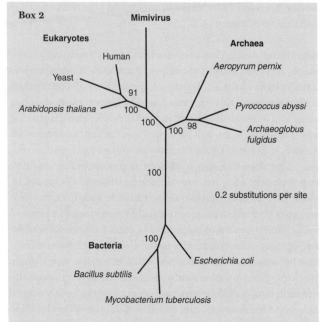

Box 2

Mimivirus

Eukaryotes

Archaea

Human

Aeropyrum pernix

Yeast

91

Arabidopsis thaliana

100

Pyrococcus abyssi

100

100 98

Archaeoglobus
fulgidus

100

0.2 substitutions per site

100

Bacteria

100

Escherichia coli

Bacillus subtilis

Mycobacterium tuberculosis

**An evolutionary tree of species from the three domains of
life showing the position of Mimivirus inferred from the gene
sequences of seven universally conserved proteins**

Viruses

glimpse this underwater menagerie, and find clues suggesting that it
plays a vital role in maintaining life on Earth. Of course, many
marine viruses cause diseases in marine animals and in so doing
pose a real threat to commercial enterprises and conservation
projects. Examples here include the highly infectious and lethal
white spot syndrome virus that has devastated shrimp farms around
the world and the turtle papillomavirus that is threatening
endangered wild turtle populations. Other viruses, such as the flu
viruses that infect seals and sea birds as well as humans, move
between land and sea and thereby facilitate transcontinental spread.

However, recent findings indicate that marine viruses also have hidden effects on the marine environment and these have profoundly influenced our view of ecology, evolution, and geochemical cycles. Plankton, which forms the oceans' floating population, consists of tiny organisms including viruses, bacteria, archaea, and eukarya. Although apparently drifting aimlessly with the sea currents, it is now clear that this population is highly structured, forming interdependent marine communities and ecosystems.

The phytoplankton is a group of organisms that uses solar energy and carbon dioxide to generate energy by photosynthesis. As a by-product of this reaction, they produce almost half of the world's oxygen and are therefore of vital importance to the chemical stability of the planet. Phytoplankton forms the base of the whole marine food-web, being grazed upon by zooplankton and young marine animals which in turn fall prey to fish and higher marine carnivores. By infecting and killing plankton microbes, marine viruses control the dynamics of all these essential populations and their interactions. For example, the common and rather beautiful phytoplankton *Emiliania huxleyi* regularly undergoes blooms that turn the ocean surface an opaque blue over areas so vast that they can be detected from space by satellites. These blooms disappear as quickly as they arise, and this boom-and-bust cycle is orchestrated by the viruses in the community that specifically infect *E. huxleyi*. Because they can produce thousands of offspring from every infected cell, virus numbers amplify in a matter of hours and so act as a rapid-response team, killing most of the bloom microbes in just a few days.

The majority of marine viruses are phages which infect and control marine bacteria populations. But that is not all they do. Phages are well known for mistakenly incorporating bits of DNA from one host and carrying them to the next, thereby spreading genetic material rapidly between their host bacteria. In the marine environment, this behaviour, which has been referred to as 'viral sex', seems to be rife, with viruses capturing host genes and passing them around the community. In this random process, captured genes will only rarely be useful to their new host, but when they are, they can become surprisingly common. They may, for example, assist their hosts in adapting rapidly to changes in nutrient levels or extreme conditions such as the high temperatures, pressures, and chemical concentrations found at deep sea vents, so allowing them to colonize a new niche.

As well as acting as mobile gene banks, some phages carry genes that give a metabolic boost to their prey. For example, many cyanophages that infect cyanobacteria, the only bacterial members of the phytoplankton, carry their own photosynthetic genes. These genes counteract the effect of other viral genes that are designed to shut down host genes in order to produce viral rather than host proteins. But inhibiting photosynthesis too early would cut the cell's life line and prevent completion of the virus life cycle, so cyanophages supply the key components of the process. These viruses have spread their photosynthesis genes so widely that now

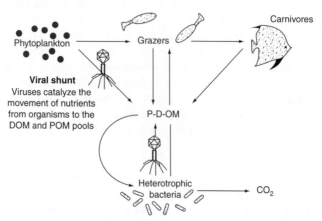

DOM = dissolved organic matter
POM = particulate organic matter

5. A diagram of biogeochemical cycling showing the viral shunt

an estimated 10% of the world's photosynthesis is carried out by genes that came from cyanophages.

As the phytoplankton requires sunlight to generate energy, these microbes inhabit the upper layers of the ocean, but viruses have no such restrictions. There are around 10^6 different viral species in a kilogram of marine sediment where they infect and kill co-resident bacteria. Overall, marine viruses kill an estimated 20–40% of marine bacteria every day, and as the major killer of marine microbes, they profoundly affect the carbon cycle by the so-called 'viral shunt' (Figure 5).

By killing other microbes, viruses convert their biomass into particulate and dissolved organic carbon that is reused by microbial communities. This increases their viability and carbon dioxide production at the expense of those higher up the food web. Without this viral shunt, much of the particulate organic carbon would sink and be sequestered on the sea bed. The net effect of this viral activity is to release around 650 million tonnes of carbon globally per year (the burning of fossil fuel is said to release around 21.3 billion tonnes of carbon dioxide per year), so contributing significantly to the build-up of carbon dioxide in the atmosphere.

Although it is now clear that the oceans are host to multitudes of viruses, we have only just begun to explore this vast reservoir. With the discovery of the abundance and diversity of marine viruses, it is likely that similar reservoirs exist in other microbial haunts, such as the human gut, where there are so many bacteria that in the body overall they outnumber human cells by 12 to 1. Despite their tiny size, viruses are proving to be of prime importance in the stability of ecosystems worldwide.

Back on dry land, viruses have also been discovered performing amazing feats. Recently, their direct role in an apparently simple symbiotic relationship between a bacterium and its host has been uncovered. Many invertebrate species carry symbiotic bacteria which may supply nutrients lacking in the animals' diet or protect them from natural predators. One such is the pea aphid, *Acyrthosiphon pisum*, which carries bacteria that protect it from the parasitic wasp, *Aphidius ervi*, that lays its eggs in the aphid haemocoel (a blood-filled space). Without this bacterium, *Hamiltonella defensa*, the aphids die as the wasp larvae develop, but toxins produced by the bacteria kill the developing wasps. The twist in the story came with the recent discovery that it is actually a phage that infects *H. defensa* that produces the wasp-killing toxin. Thus three very different organisms work together to combat their mutual enemy: the parasitic wasp.

A similar story relates to *Vibrio cholerae*, the cause of cholera in humans. This bacterium resides in the waters of the Ganges Delta alongside a variety of phage strains that infect it. Some of these phages kill the bacterium (lytic phage) and others carry the cholera toxin gene (toxigenic phage). Only cholera bacteria infected with the toxigenic phage are pathogenic to humans, causing the devastating and often fatal diarrhoea of cholera.

A cholera epidemic usually begins during the wet season when the river swells, so diluting the phage concentration and allowing the cholera vibrios to multiply (Figure 6). People drinking the river water will ingest a mixture of vibrios with and without toxigenic phage, but only the toxigenic vibrios survive and multiply inside the human gut. These cause terrible stomach cramps and copious watery diarrhoea, which not only leads to rapid dehydration but also extrudes thousands of toxigenic microbes back into the environment. Thus the concentration of toxigenic vibrios rises, which fuels the epidemic. But this also results in a population explosion among the lytic phages that feed on *V. cholerae*. Eventually, the lytic phages control the toxigenic bacteria and the natural balance is resumed, until heavy rains again destabilize the situation.

A chapter on the ubiquity of viruses is not complete without discussing the possibility that viruses exist in outer space. Of

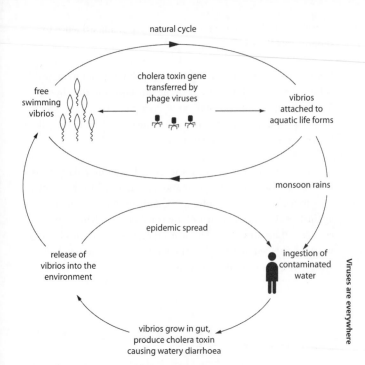

natural cycle

cholera toxin gene transferred by phage viruses

free swimming vibrios

vibrios attached to aquatic life forms

monsoon rains

epidemic spread

release of vibrios into the environment

ingestion of contaminated water

vibrios grow in gut, produce cholera toxin causing watery diarrhoea

Viruses are everywhere

6. The cholera cycle, showing the natural cycle and the epidemic spread that can occur after the monsoon rains

course, viruses, as obligate parasites, can only exist where life is found, so the question becomes, is there any life, microbial or otherwise, on other planets? At present, we don't know the answer to this, although in the 1970s Sir Fred Hoyle, famous astronomer and sci-fi writer, conceived the theory of 'panspermia'. This states that life on Earth began with bacteria and viruses seeded from outer space via comets. Hoyle and his followers believed that these microbes continue to arrive today, so contributing to microbe evolution and emerging infections. Apparently, the interior of a comet would provide the warm, damp conditions required for microbes to thrive. Be that as it may, exhaustive searches of material from Mars have produced no convincing evidence to support this theory.

Water is a basic requirement for life as we know it. Many scientists believe that, given the vastness of the universe, and the almost inconceivable number of stars in it, there must be life out there somewhere. If there is life, then the chances are that there will be viruses as well, but we shall just have to wait and see.

In the next chapter, we look at the battle fought on a daily basis between viruses and their plant and animal hosts. In this struggle for survival, hosts have evolved mechanisms to protect themselves against viral attack, but viruses are constantly evolving new counter-attack strategies. This arms race, ongoing over millions of years, has helped to drive the sophistication of the human immune system and has ensured our survival.

Chapter 3
Kill or be killed

Viruses parasitize all living things, often to the detriment of their hosts, but they do not have it all their own way. All plants and animals, however small or primitive, have evolved ways of recognizing and fighting these microscopic invaders. So for most viruses, each round of infection is a race against time – they must reproduce before the host either dies or its immune system recognizes and eliminates them. Then their offspring must find new hosts to infect and repeat the process *ad infinitum* in order for the species to survive. Even viruses that have learned the trick of dodging immune attack and live happily inside their host for its lifetime must eventually move on to avoid dying with the host.

The success of this precarious lifestyle critically depends on viruses spreading efficiently between susceptible hosts, and yet this is a process that viruses have to leave entirely to chance as their particles are completely inert. Add to this the fact that after infection with a particular virus all vertebrates, and several more primitive organisms, are immune to re-infection, it seems surprising that viruses can survive at all.

Viruses endure because they are so adaptable. Their fast reproduction rate and large number of offspring means that they can evolve rapidly to meet changing circumstances. No doubt many virus species *have* died out when their routes of spread were

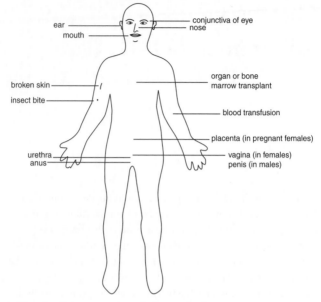

7. Portals of virus entry into the human body

blocked but, at the same time, others will have found new routes opening up and seized the opportunity to flourish. Thus virus populations are highly dynamic, with one rapidly replacing another if its 'fitness' best suits the prevailing climate. We have seen how, for example, the present measles virus strain replaced its ancestor globally around 200 years ago, and how populations of marine phage viruses are constantly changing depending on the advantage they can gain by stealing genes from their hosts.

Viruses spread between hosts by almost every conceivable route (Figure 7). Those that can survive outside their host for a period of time may travel through the air, like flu, measles, and common cold viruses, or by contaminating food and water like noro- and rotaviruses that can cause massive outbreaks of diarrhoea and vomiting, particularly where standards of hygiene are low.

By constantly evolving, these viruses appear to have honed their skills for spreading from one host to another to reach an amazing degree of sophistication. For example, the common cold virus (rhinovirus), while infecting cells lining the nasal cavities, tickles nerve endings, a process that causes sneezing. During these 'explosions', huge clouds of virus-carrying mucus droplets are forcefully ejected, then float in the air until inhaled by other susceptible hosts. Similarly, by wiping out sheets of cells lining the intestine, rotavirus prevents the absorption of fluids from the gut cavity. This causes severe diarrhoea and vomiting that effectively extrudes the virus's offspring back into the environment to reach new hosts.

Other highly successful viruses hitch a ride from one host to another with insects. Plant viruses may be spread by aphids that tap into the plant's sap, and in the same way biting insects suck viruses up from one host and inject them into another while taking a blood meal. Examples include dengue fever virus and yellow fever virus, both of which are ferried between hosts by female mosquitoes that require a blood meal to nourish their eggs. These viruses cause very large epidemics in tropical and subtropical areas where their particular host mosquito species live.

Viruses cannot infect the outer, dead layers of our skin, or penetrate through the multiple layers of intact skin, but a microscopic abrasion is enough to allow entry of wart (papilloma) and cold sore (herpes simplex) viruses, both very common infections caught directly from an infected host. But viruses that are too fragile to live for long outside their host's body may be passed directly from one to another through close contact such as kissing. This is a very effective way of transmitting viruses in saliva, like Epstein–Barr virus which causes glandular fever, also known as 'the kissing disease'. Some viruses like HIV and hepatitis B (HBV) make use of the sexual route of transmission, particularly when other sexually transmitted microbes, such as *Gonococcus* and *Treponema pallidum* (the cause of syphilis), provide easy access by producing surface ulceration. These viruses also exploit modern interventions like surgical instruments, dentists' drills, blood transfusion, and organ transplantation to jump from one host to another. Indeed, HBV is so highly infectious that a microscopic amount of blood is enough to transmit the infection, making it a serious occupational hazard for healthcare workers in contact with HBV-infected people.

All living organisms have defences against invading viruses. Although this protective immunity is most highly developed in vertebrates, reaching a peak of sophistication in humans, we now know that even the simplest of organisms have immune mechanisms, many of which are very different from those found in vertebrates. We are still a long way from understanding the extent and details of these mechanisms, but new information is continually emerging. It used to be thought that only vertebrates have immunological memory, but studies on repeat host exposure to the same pathogen now indicate that even in some primitive invertebrates the first infection provides some protection from a subsequent one, suggesting that some basic memory response exists in lower life forms.

Another recently discovered protective mechanism, first identified in plants but also used by insects and other animal species, is gene silencing by RNA interference (RNAi). Interfering RNAs are short RNA molecules that are found inside cells of most species, including humans, where they regulate the manufacture of proteins by binding to RNA messages and preventing their translation into protein. When a virus infects a cell and commandeers its protein-manufacturing processes, RNAi molecules also bind to viral RNA messages and inhibit their translation into proteins, so aborting the infection before new viruses can be assembled. A similar but novel immune mechanism related to RNAi has recently come to light in archaea and bacteria, helping them to combat phage attack. In this system, short gene segments from invading phages are incorporated into the host genome. These then code for RNAs which specifically bind the invader's proteins and inhibit subsequent protein production, so aborting the infection before new viruses can be assembled.

Clearly, the battle between humans and microbes has been ongoing ever since humans evolved, with microbes evolving new means of attack and our immune system retaliating with improved defences in an escalating arms race. As a virus's generation time is so much shorter than ours, the evolution of genetic resistance to a new human virus is painfully slow, and constantly leaves viruses in the driving seat.

A recent example of genetic resistance was uncovered during research to discover why some people were apparently resistant to HIV infection. This turned out to be related to an immune response gene called CCR5 that codes for a protein that is essential for HIV infection. About 10% of the Caucasian population has a deletion in this gene that confers resistance to HIV infection. How the deletion reached such a high level in this human population remains a mystery. Although the CCR5 deletion happens to block HIV infection, humans were infected with HIV far too recently to have produced this effect, since it takes many generations for a gene mutation to reach such a high level over a broad geographical area, in this case throughout Europe and Asia. Scientists think that the CCR5 deletion must have conferred a selective advantage in the past by protecting against a lethal microbe, with plague and smallpox being strong contenders as they have both been major killers for over 2,000 years.

The human immune system is a fearsome fighting machine that uses two modes of operation, a non-specific, rapid-response mode and a slower, but highly specific killing force that remembers the attacker and prevents it from breaching the body's defences again. Viruses often gain access to the body by infecting cells of the respiratory, intestinal, or genitourinary tracts, the deeper layers of the skin, and the surface of the eye, and may then disseminate from these areas to infect internal organs. At the primary site of infection, cells send out chemical signals, called cytokines. Most important of these early signals is interferon, which renders surrounding cells resistant to infection at the same time as alerting the immune system to start an attack by attracting its component cells to the area. Amoeba-like cells called polymorphs and macrophages are the first to arrive on the scene, where they gobble up viruses and virus-infected cells as well as pump out more cytokines to attract the lymphocyte contingents, an essential part of the human immune response. Traditionally, these are termed B and T lymphocytes based on the type of immune response they elicit.

Each part of the body is protected by lymph glands that act as garrisons for millions of B and T lymphocytes. The tonsils and adenoids, for example, are strategically placed around the entrances to the respiratory and intestinal tracts, and similar glands in the groin, armpit, and neck protect the legs, arms, and head respectively. Virus-chomping macrophages make their way from the site of infection to these local lymph glands where they display chopped-up viral proteins to the B and T lymphocytes to engender a specific immune response.

Individual B and T lymphocytes carry unique receptors that only recognize one small segment of a particular protein, called an antigen. To cover all possible microbe antigens, our bodies contain around 2×10^{12} of both B and T lymphocytes that circulate in our blood and are constantly replenished from the blood cell factory in our bone marrow. Lymphocytes congregate in lymph glands waiting for their wake-up call in the form of a macrophage bearing an antigen that exactly fits their unique receptor. When this finally comes, the union of receptor and antigen stimulates the lymphocyte to divide rapidly, forming a clone of cells with identical receptors. These are generally ready for action about a week after the initial infection.

T lymphocytes (or T cells) are the body's single most important defence against viruses. There are two main types of T cells: helper T cells, characterized by the CD4 molecule on their surface, and killer (or cytotoxic) T cells, characterized by the CD8 molecule. Both CD4 and CD8 T cells kill virus-infected cells through the production of toxic chemicals that rupture the cell membrane, and CD4 T cells also produce cytokines that help CD8 T cells and B lymphocytes to grow, mature, and function properly.

Once B lymphocytes (or B cells) are galvanized into action by their specific antigen, they make antibodies, which are soluble molecules that circulate in the blood, and pass into tissues and onto body surfaces such as the lining of the gut. Antibodies bind to viruses and virus-infected cells, helping to prevent spread of the invaders. In some instances, antibodies actually prevent viruses from infecting cells by blocking their receptor for entry and therefore are important in preventing later re-infection.

The relative importance of T and B cells in the control of virus infections is well illustrated by rare mutations that wipe out one or other lymphocyte type. Babies born with a mutation that eliminates their T cells die very rapidly of virus infections unless they live inside a germ-free bubble until they get a bone marrow transplant to correct the defect. Alternatively, babies with a mutation that prevents B cell development cope fairly well with virus infections but suffer from severe and persistent bacterial and fungal infections. However, they are generally protected from these infections during the first few months of life (as are healthy babies) by antibodies from their mother's blood that cross the placenta in late pregnancy and are also present in breast milk.

The immune response to microbes is a complex but finely balanced operation, with the action of cells fighting the invaders counterbalanced by a group of cells called regulatory T cells. These produce cytokines that defuse a T cell's killing mechanism and stop it dividing, so that once the microbe is defeated, the fighting cells die and the response is brought to an end, leaving only a skeleton crew of memory T and B cells ready for rapid action when the microbe appears again.

At the height of its activity, the immune response may be so pronounced that it actually does harm to the body. In fact, the typical, non-specific symptoms we experience with an acute dose of flu, such as fever, headache, enlarged tender glands, and general fatigue, are often not caused by the invading microbe itself but by the cytokines released by immune cells to fight it. On rare occasions, these immune-induced reactions may cause serious injury to internal organs, a result known as immunopathology. Examples include liver damage during infection with hepatitis viruses and the severe fatigue experienced by sufferers of glandular fever caused by Epstein–Barr virus. Alternatively, T cells or antibodies specific for viral proteins may, by chance, recognize, or cross-react with, a similar host protein. This can lead to damage to, or the death of, cells expressing the protein. This autoimmune process may be the basis of diseases such as diabetes, in which the insulin-producing beta cells in the pancreas are destroyed, and multiple sclerosis that results from destruction of cells in the central nervous system.

Some viruses have learned to play hide-and-seek with immune cells by protecting themselves from the ensuing onslaught and remaining in their host for long periods, even for life. Strategies employed by these viruses are as varied as they are ingenious, including evasion of immune recognition and/or obstruction of the immune response. Details of these are discussed in Chapter 6, but suffice it to say that each step of the immune cascade, from the initial interferon release to the killer T cell attack and the later calming action of regulatory T cells, can be modified by one virus or another to promote their own survival.

For instance, HIV has several means of immune evasion including integration of its provirus into the host cell genome where it masquerades as a piece of host DNA. But in this state, the virus is still potentially exposed to immune attack when it replicates. To evade this, HIV mutates rapidly, changing the composition of its surface proteins to avoid recognition by specific T cells and antibodies. HIV also infects and destroys CD4 T cells, the very cells that drive the immune response against it. So as the infection progresses and the host's immunity weakens, the virus can multiply in the body unchecked along with other 'opportunistic' microbes that the body can no longer control.

Most viruses induce solid immunity so that once recovered from an infection the host is resistant to further attack by the same virus. This naturally occurring immunity is mimicked by vaccines which may consist of killed or modified whole virus, or part of a virus. This tricks the immune system into responding as if to a natural infection, thus preventing any later attack. The various ways vaccines have been developed and used to prevent devastating viral diseases and even completely eradicate pathogenic viruses are described in Chapter 8.

Chapter 4
Emerging virus infections

Emerging infections engender fear sometimes verging on panic as an unknown microbe appears without warning, infecting and killing populations, apparently indiscriminately. Although this scenario is more often the subject of horror movies than real life, the fact remains that today 'new' microbes are emerging with increasing frequency (Figure 8). Indeed, the first outbreak of SARS in 2003 and the swine flu pandemic in 2009 were very worrying until scientists discovered the cause and worked out control strategies.

In this chapter, the term 'emerging virus infection' refers to both the emergence of an infectious disease caused by a virus that is entirely new to the species it infects, and to a re-emerging infection, meaning that the disease is increasing in frequency, either in its traditional geographic location or in a new area. Obvious examples of the former include swine flu and bird flu, as well as SARS coronavirus, all of which infected and spread among humans for the first time recently. A good example of a re-emerging infection is West Nile virus, which emerged on the eastern seaboard of the USA in 1999, having arrived from Israel, and then crossed the entire continent in just four years. Newly discovered viruses which cause well-established diseases are also sometimes referred to as emerging infections. These include

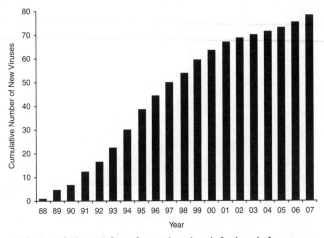

8. The cumulative number of emerging virus infections in humans from 1988 to 2007

some tumour viruses, not mentioned in this chapter as they are covered in Chapter 6.

Novel viruses that emerge and spread successfully in a naïve host population produce an epidemic, defined as 'an infection occurring at a higher than expected frequency', and may progress to a pandemic if it is spreading on several continents at once. However, these definitions give no indication of the extent or duration of a disease outbreak. The differing patterns of emerging infectious disease outbreaks depend on a number of viral factors, including its incubation period and method of spread, and important host behavioural factors like living conditions, propensity to travel, and the success of any preventive measures. Both HIV and SARS emerged fairly recently, but the pattern of these outbreaks couldn't have been more different. Whereas the SARS epidemic was short and sharp, all over in a few months (Figure 9), the HIV pandemic has lasted decades and is still ongoing (Figure 10).

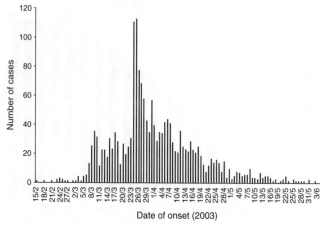

9. The emergence of SARS in Hong Kong. The figure shows the number of new cases per day from February to June 2003

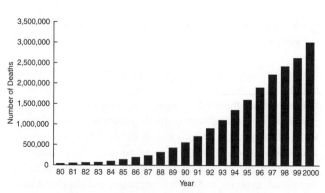

10. The estimated number of AIDS-related deaths worldwide from 1980 to 2000

SARS coronavirus first emerged in November 2002 in Foshan, Guangdong Province, China, where it caused an outbreak of atypical pneumonia. Initially, the virus spread locally, particularly among patients' family members and hospital staff, but everything changed in February 2003 when a doctor who had treated SARS cases in Guangdong Province unwittingly carried the virus to Hong Kong. He stayed one night at the Metropole Hotel in Hong Kong before being admitted to hospital, where he died of SARS a few days later. In the hospital, the virus spread to staff, which sparked the Hong Kong epidemic. During his 24-hour stay in the hotel, the doctor transmitted the virus to at least 17 guests (apparently he sneezed in the lift), who then carried it to 5 more countries, thus spawning epidemics in Canada, Vietnam, and Singapore. This rapid dissemination of the virus threatened to cause a pandemic, but surprisingly by July 2003 it was over, the final toll being around 8,000 cases and 800 deaths involving 29 countries across 5 continents.

SARS coronavirus spreads through the air and causes disease in almost everyone it infects. After an incubation period of 2 to 14 days, victims develop fever, malaise, muscle aches, and a cough, sometimes progressing rapidly to viral pneumonia that requires intensive care, with mechanical ventilation in around 20% of cases. But with no known treatment or preventive vaccine, how was the epidemic conquered so effectively?

Left to its own devices, SARS coronavirus would undoubtedly have continued its trail of destruction but, fortunately, many of its characteristics played into the hands of those trying to stop it, and contributed to its speedy demise. Importantly, the virus mostly causes overt disease, with few unidentified silent infections. This meant that cases and their contacts could be recognized and isolated, and since victims are only infectious once the symptoms have developed, this prevented further spread. Also, as the disease is usually severe and debilitating, relatively few patients, excepting the doctor from Guangdong, travelled far while infectious. During SARS, the virus is produced in the lungs and spread by coughing. This generates relatively heavy mucus droplets that do not spread far through the air; hence close contacts like family members and hospital staff are mainly at risk, the latter constituting over 20%

37

of cases worldwide. Once all these factors were appreciated, old-fashioned barrier nursing and isolation of patients and their contacts were enough to interrupt virus spread and prevent a pandemic.

Unlike SARS coronavirus, HIV has been spreading among humans since the early 1900s and despite drugs which control the infection, it is still on the increase in certain areas of the world. Currently, there are 33 million people living with HIV, and it has caused over 25 million deaths since the first report of AIDS in 1981. It is interesting to examine the reasons for this lack of control, and to contrast these with the success of the SARS control programme.

Firstly, although SARS coronavirus had spread internationally by the time it was recognized by the World Health Organization (WHO), it had only infected humans for a few months. Compare this to the estimated 100 years during which HIV was silently creeping around sub-Saharan Africa, where poverty, wars, and poor health services conspired to facilitate its spread, and prevent the recognition of AIDS as a new disease.

Secondly, in contrast to SARS' short incubation period and infectivity coinciding with overt disease, HIV has an average asymptomatic period of eight to ten years, and during this time the carrier may transmit the virus to any number of contacts.

Thirdly, the two viruses spread by completely different means. Whereas SARS coronavirus's airborne flight can easily be intercepted, interruption of HIV's transmission is more problematic. HIV spreads most commonly by sexual contact. Other routes of spread include mother to child during birth and breast feeding, in transplanted organs, transfused blood and blood products, and via contamination of surgical instruments as well as injecting drug users' equipment. These non-sexual routes can in theory be interrupted, but they are almost insignificant in global terms compared to its spread via heterosexual contact. In exploiting the basic human urge to procreate, HIV targets the young and sexually active and is passed unwittingly from one apparently healthy host to another through sexual networks. Although its transmission can be halted by barrier devices, the vast amounts of money spent on the promotion of condom use for safer sex have not altered sexual practices sufficiently to halt the pandemic.

Untreated HIV infection leads to AIDS after a lengthy silent period, and this syndrome was first recognized in 1981 in San Francisco when several gay men died of unusual infections superimposed on severe HIV-induced immunosuppression. As the extent of the pandemic became apparent, three distinct risk groups emerged: people with multiple sexual partners, both heterosexual and homosexual; people with haemophilia or other disorders requiring regular infusions of blood or blood products; and injecting drug users. Utilizing the molecular clock technique to track back to the origin of HIV in humans, sub-Saharan Africa, particularly Kinshasa in the Democratic Republic of Congo (DRC), was pinpointed as the epicentre of the pandemic. Then using two early viruses isolated from people living in DRC, scientists have calculated that HIV has infected people in this region for around 100 years. They have identified a single virus strain that carried the infection from DRC to Haiti and another that transported the infection from Haiti to the USA. So by the time HIV was discovered in 1983, the pandemic was already growing exponentially and has proved very difficult to control.

A virus that jumps to a new host species for the first time has a series of hurdles to overcome before it can establish itself in the naïve population. Firstly, it must infect cells of the new host, and this involves finding a host cell receptor molecule to lock on to. Many would-be virus infections abort at this point, a fact that explains the species barrier of most viruses. Even if the new virus can unlock and enter host cells, it still may not be able to reproduce inside them, resulting in another abortive infection. For instance,

HIV cannot infect mouse CD4 T cells because the molecular structure of the mouse CD4 molecule differs from the human equivalent in ways that make it unrecognizable to the virus. Even if mouse T cells are transplanted with the human HIV receptor molecules (CD4 and CCR5) in the laboratory, the infection is still abortive because mouse T cells lack the essential proteins that the virus requires for its replication.

However, on occasions viruses do enter and successfully replicate in cells of a new host species, but after a window of opportunity lasting about a week during which they can colonize the host and reproduce, their offspring must move on to another susceptible host before the developing host immunity wipes them out. SARS coronavirus and H5N1 (bird) flu have both managed to infect humans but differ in their success to date. Whereas SARS coronavirus can spread between humans, H5N1 flu, which first jumped from birds to humans in 1997, is unable to do so. This flu virus strain is still poorly adapted to its new (human) host, and we will be in danger of an H5N1 flu pandemic only once it evolves an efficient method of spreading between us.

Most apparently novel viruses that infect humans are not entirely new. They are either viruses that have mutated or recombined sufficiently to be unrecognizable by our immune system, or, more commonly, they have come from other animals, seizing the opportunity to hop from one animal species to another when the two come into contact. The latter are called zoonotic viruses, and the diseases they cause are zoonoses.

As we have seen, RNA viruses mutate much more frequently than DNA viruses, producing a variety of offspring, of which some can dodge host immunity more efficiently than their siblings and therefore flourish at their expense. Eventually, a virus emerges that is sufficiently different from its ancestors to be immunologically unrecognizable. Then everyone in the host population will be susceptible and it may cause an epidemic. Flu is a prime example of a virus that mutates frequently, a process called antigenic drift. The flu virus circulates constantly in the community, accumulating genetic changes and causing regular winter outbreaks and larger epidemics every eight to ten years. However, its story is actually much more complicated. There are three flu strains, A, B, and C, and flu A is a zoonotic virus. With the help of wild birds, this virus can also undergo recombination, or antigenic shift, producing an entirely new strain of flu in one go by exchanging fragments of its genome with other strains. This has the potential to cause a pandemic.

The natural hosts of flu A viruses are aquatic birds, particularly ducks, but the viruses also infect a variety of other animals including domestic poultry, pigs, horses, cats, and seals. Flu A replicates in birds' guts and is excreted in their faeces, causing no symptoms but effectively spreading to other bird populations. Flu viruses have eight genes which are segmented, meaning that instead of its genome being a continuous strand of RNA, each gene forms a separate strand. The H (haemaglutinin) and N (neuraminidase) genes are the most important in stimulating protective host immunity. There are 16 different H and 9 different N genes, all of which can be found in all combinations in bird flu viruses. Because these genes are separate RNA strands in the virus, on occasions they become mixed up, or recombined. So if two flu A viruses with different H and/or N genes infect a single cell, the offspring will carry varying combinations of genes from the two parent viruses. Most of these viruses will not be able to infect humans, but occasionally a new virus strain is produced that can jump directly to humans and cause a pandemic, as we have experienced recently with swine flu.

Over the last century, there have been five flu pandemics: in the H1N1 'Spanish' flu of 1918, all eight genes came from birds; the H2N2 'Asian' flu of 1957 acquired three new genes, including H and N from birds; and the H3N2 'Hong Kong' flu of 1968 acquired two new genes from wild ducks. The 'Russian' flu of 1977, which probably escaped from a lab in Russia, was a 1950s version of H1N1; whereas the H1N1 'swine' flu which appeared in Mexico in 2009 has six genes from North American and two genes from Eurasian pig flu viruses.

On average, flu A epidemics and pandemics kill around one in a thousand of those infected, with the very young, the very old, and those with chronic diseases being particularly at risk. Pandemics additionally often target young adults: in the 1977 Russian flu pandemic, the young were hardest hit because they had no previous immunity, whereas most older people were spared as they were already immune. Similarly, in the recent swine flu pandemic the disease was most severe in young adults and pregnant women. However, by far the most virulent flu virus on record is the 1918 pandemic strain which targeted young adults and killed 40–50 million people worldwide, around 2.5% of all those infected.

With the virulent H5N1 bird flu on the horizon, the late 1990s saw a flurry of activity aimed at finding out why the H1N1, 1918 flu was so deadly. Amazingly, researchers managed to reconstruct the virus using samples taken from a flu victim buried in the permafrost in Alaska, and from post-mortem lung samples from a US serviceman stored in a pathology laboratory for some 80 years. Compared to non-pandemic H1N1 virus, the 1918 strain has several mutations that enhance its infectivity and growth rate in human cells. In particular, a mutation in a gene called NS1 prevents virus-infected cells from producing interferon, the key cytokine for preventing virus spread and triggering the whole immune cascade. This allows the virus to get a head start, and in some cases the body responds with an uncontrolled outpouring of cytokines, called a cytokine storm. A massive and inappropriate inflammatory response ensues that may cause death from respiratory failure as the victim's lungs fill with fluid. This mutation is already present in the H5N1 bird flu virus, accounting for the high mortality rate among those it infects. Fortunately, it has not learned to spread between humans so far.

The transfer of 'new' zoonotic viruses from their primary host to humans can be facilitated by certain behaviours or cultural practices, and we now know that a particular risk is our interaction with wild animals, many of which carry viruses with the potential to infect us. Both HIV and SARS coronavirus were introduced into the human population when their natural hosts were hunted and killed for consumption.

It is now clear that HIV-like viruses have jumped from primates to humans in central Africa on several occasions and that one of these viruses, HIV-1 type M, has succeeded in spreading globally. The ancestor of this virus has been traced to a subspecies of chimpanzees (*Pan troglodytes troglodytes*), among whom it can cause an AIDS-like disease. Since these animals are hunted for bush meat, it is most likely that human infection occurred by blood contamination during the killing and butchering process. This transfer took place some 100 years ago, probably in southeast Cameroon where the chimpanzees carrying the virus most similar to HIV-1 type M live. Scientists postulate that the virus (inside humans) travelled from Cameroon along the Sangha River, a tributary of the Congo River, to reach Leopoldville (now called Kinshasa), then the capital of the former Belgian Congo, from where it spread globally.

SARS coronavirus also entered the human population from an animal food source, this time in the live animal markets of China. Here, there are a number of small mammals on offer and several, most noticeably the Himalayan palm civet cat, carry SARS-like viruses. As the natural reservoir of SARS coronavirus has now been identified as the fruit bat, it is presumed that the virus transferred to other animal species in markets where they are packed into overcrowded cages, and then jumped to the market traders.

SARS is not the only potentially lethal virus carried by bats; several bat species are reservoirs for viruses that have recently jumped to humans. In fact, bats almost certainly transmit the much-feared and highly infectious Ebola and Ebola-like viruses. Epidemics of Ebola viral haemorrhagic fever hit rural populations in central Africa from time to time, and these outbreaks have increased in frequency in DRC, Gabon, and Sudan since the mid-1990s. Ebola virus was discovered after an explosive outbreak in Yambuku, a remote village in northern Zaire (now DRC), in 1976, and was named after the local Ebola River. This epidemic began with a school teacher who developed a headache and fever after returning from a trip into the bush. He was treated for malaria at the local mission hospital, but his symptoms progressed to a full-blown viral haemorrhagic fever with soaring temperature, severe abdominal pain, diarrhoea, vomiting, muscle cramps, and generalized bleeding. He died within a few days. The virus, transmitted by direct contact with the patient and his body fluids, then spread to his family, other hospital patients, and staff, eventually infecting 318 people in the village and killing 280 of them.

Counter-intuitively, control of Ebola outbreaks is quite straightforward once the disease is recognized. Since the infection is so debilitating, few infected victims move far from the outbreak site, and once the person-to-person chain of infection is broken by strict barrier nursing and isolation of cases and contacts, it can be rapidly controlled. Unfortunately, the virus has recently jumped to large apes, particularly chimpanzees and lowland gorillas. This not only threatens the very existence of these endangered species, but also provides an additional transmission route to humans when they come into contact with these animals, perhaps accounting for the recent reported rise in outbreaks.

Another dangerous bat-transmitted virus emerged in 1997 when a group of Malaysian farmers reported a respiratory disease outbreak among their pigs, and later several pig farmers and abattoir workers came down with encephalitis. Fortunately, the disease did not spread directly from person to person, and was later controlled by slaughtering over a million pigs in 1999. Sadly, by this time, there had been 265 cases of encephalitis with 105 fatalities. A novel paramyxovirus was isolated from a victim's brain and named Nipah virus after the village in which he lived. The virus was traced to fruit bats, and its trail to humans probably began when a colony of bats was left homeless by deforestation. The bats relocated to trees near the pig farms and the virus spread to the pigs via bat droppings, and then from the pigs to the farmers and abattoir workers.

Due to our invasion of their territories, bats and humans are coming into contact with increasing frequency. The Nipah virus turns out to be very similar to bat-borne Hendra virus, isolated in 1994 from the victims of an outbreak of severe respiratory disease on Hendra farm in Brisbane, Australia, where it killed 14 horses and one of their trainers. Similar outbreaks in West Bengal in 2001 and in Bangladesh in 2001 and 2004 are also attributed to bat viruses, indicating that these cute, furry animals are far from safe companions.

Several insect species act as virus vectors, ferrying them from one host to another, so that any changes in vector population density directly affect transmission of these viruses. Ever since 2004, when the use of the insecticide DDT (dichloro-diphenyl-trichloroethane) was restricted by the Stockholm Convention on Persistent Organic Pollutants, mosquitoes in certain tropical and subtropical areas have undergone a population explosion. This has led to the re-emergence of several mosquito-borne microbes, including dengue virus. Traditionally restricted to South-East Asia, dengue virus has been spreading to new geographical areas for the last 60 years, and is now a major problem in tropical Africa and South America (Figure 11).

Dengue virus often infects without causing symptoms, but it may cause classical dengue fever, characterized by a rising temperature; severe headache; muscle, bone, and joint pains; vomiting; and a skin rash. For obvious reasons, the disease is dubbed 'break-bone fever', but although unpleasant, full recovery is the rule. However,

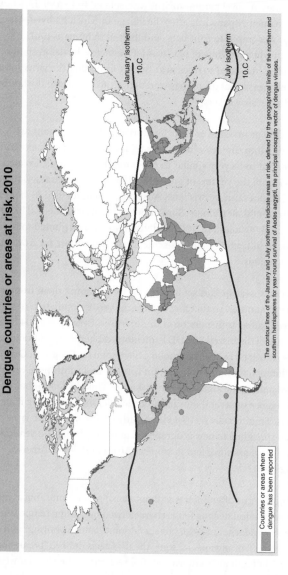

Dengue, countries or areas at risk, 2010

January isotherm
10.C

July isotherm
10.C

The contour lines of the January and July isotherms indicate areas at risk, defined by the geographical limits of the northern and southern hemispheres for year-round survival of Aedes aegypti, the principal mosquito vector of dengue viruses.

Countries or areas where
dengue has been reported

11. The worldwide distribution of dengue fever in 2010

in 1–2% of cases this progresses to dengue haemorrhagic fever, with bleeding into the skin, gastrointestinal tract, and lungs leading to circulatory failure – called dengue shock syndrome. With no specific treatment, the syndrome has a high mortality.

Bluetongue virus is another insect-borne microbe that has socioeconomic consequences since it infects domestic animals, mainly sheep, and is spread between them by midges. Once infected, sheep develop fever followed by excessive salivation, frothing at the mouth, nasal discharge, and swelling of the face and tongue. The bluish tinge to the sheep's tongue, caused by low blood oxygen levels, gives the disease its name. Lameness is another symptom, and pneumonia may develop which can prove fatal. More often, a slow recovery ensues, but impairment of wool growth is an important commercial consequence.

Bluetongue was first recorded in South Africa and has traditionally been restricted to tropical and subtropical areas where it also infects cattle and goats, although with milder symptoms than in sheep. Its geographical distribution reflects the fact that African midges cannot survive severe winters. However, thanks to global warming, the midge has recently extended its territory into southern Europe, where the virus has been picked up by hardier European midges. Each year, the insects undergo a population explosion in early summer, when transmission of bluetongue virus peaks. Bluetongue has been moving steadily northwards and was recorded in Germany, France, Holland, and Belgium in 2006 where it survived the winter, and reached the UK and Denmark in 2007, Sweden in 2008, and Norway in 2009. So will the midge's unwelcome passenger virus survive these northern climes, become indigenous, and affect domestic animals? Only time will tell.

With these examples of emerging and re-emerging infections in mind, we can now address the question of why they are presently on the rise in both humans and domestic animals.

Many modern-day lifestyle factors increase our risk of emerging infections, and most of these are linked to overpopulation. The world's population approximately doubled every 500 years between the beginning of the Christian era and 1900, when it reached 1.6 billion. But in the 20th century, life expectancy rose steeply and the population quadrupled, hitting 6 billion by 2000. If this growth rate continues unabated, we are set to reach 9 to 10 billion by 2100.

A population of this size brings many problems, not least diminishing natural resources, increasing pollution, loss of biodiversity, and global warming. But as far as emerging virus infections are concerned, the most acute problem is literally lack of space. We have already seen how invading the territories of wild animals, be it to chop down the rain forest, hunt for food, or extend our cities, risks acquiring unknown, sometimes lethal, viruses. With over 50% of us now living in megacities, like Tokyo with over 35 million inhabitants, viruses, once acquired, find it very easy to spread between us. This is particularly so among poor city dwellers in resource-poor countries, with the inhabitants of shanty towns living in cramped, unhygienic shacks where the lack of fresh air and clean water, and absence of sewage disposal, provides easy access for microbes of all sorts. As illustrated by HIV, SARS, and swine flu, successful local spread soon leads to international dissemination. With over a billion people worldwide boarding international flights every year, novel viruses have an efficient mechanism for reaching the other side of the world within 24 hours.

Animal viruses also thrive on overpopulation. For them, intensively farmed animals equate to crowded cities and present the opportunity to spread easily among their hosts. A dramatic example is the foot and mouth disease virus outbreak in Britain in 2001 when pyres of slaughtered farm animals were seen all over the countryside. The virus, which is highly infectious among cattle, sheep, pigs, goats, and deer, is widespread in Asia, Continental Europe, Africa, and South America, but generally absent from Australasia, the USA, Canada, and the UK. It targets the skin around the mouth and hooves, leading to lameness, and although not usually fatal, the loss of condition it produces in infected animals is very economically damaging.

Animal viruses usually cross international boundaries unnoticed inside their hosts, and sometimes jump to humans on arrival at their new destination. As we have already seen, West Nile fever virus jumped from Israel to the US in 1999, although its mode of transport remains a mystery. The virus naturally infects birds and is spread among them by mosquitoes, which can then infect humans via a bite. The infection is usually asymptomatic but may cause a flu-like illness and, very occasionally, encephalitis. To date, the virus has not passed from person to person (except reportedly in a blood transfusion and a transplanted heart), so human infection is generally a dead end for the virus. This being the case, the virus must have hitched a ride to the US inside a continent-hopping bird or mosquito, and then found native US mosquitoes ready to pass it between local birds when it arrived.

No such mystery surrounds the sudden arrival of monkey pox virus in the US in 2003. Contrary to its name, this virus naturally infects African rodents and occasionally jumps to humans, causing fever, sore throat, swollen glands, and a prominent, smallpox-like rash. Fortunately, the disease is generally not life-threatening, although the rash may leave scars reminiscent of smallpox. The US outbreak, causing over 70 cases before it was controlled, was traced to imported giant Gambian rats from Ghana. In a pet shop, these rats were housed alongside prairie dogs that caught the virus and passed it on to their new owners.

This example highlights the risks involved in jetting animals around the world as part of the international trade in pets. We know little enough about microbes living in domestic animals let alone those in wild animals. It is clearly important to learn more about these reservoirs of viruses, many of which may adapt quickly to a new naïve population and could prove lethal.

Chapter 5
Epidemics and pandemics

Once an acute emerging virus such as a new strain of flu is successfully established in a population, it generally settles into a mode of cyclical epidemics during which many susceptible people are infected and become immune to further attack. When most are immune, the virus moves on, only returning when a new susceptible population has emerged, which generally consists of infants born since the last epidemic. Before vaccination programmes became widespread, young children suffered from a series of well-recognized infectious diseases called the 'childhood infections'. These included measles, mumps, rubella, and chickenpox, all caused by viruses, of which only chickenpox remains widespread in the West today.

To find out when and how humans first experienced these acute childhood infections, we need to look back some 10,000 years to the farming revolution that began in the Fertile Crescent (the area between the Rivers Tigris and Euphrates, in modern-day Iraq and Iran) and spread rapidly to neighbouring lands. This dramatic alteration in lifestyle, which was later adopted independently in several other parts of the world, converted our ancestors from nomadic hunter-gatherers to farmers living in fixed communities. The consequences of this change with respect to the microbes that infected them were equally dramatic. It led to a period of ever-increasing epidemics of severe and often lethal infections caused by microbes, including those that we now recognize among the acute childhood illnesses.

This onslaught was directly related to the change in lifestyle. Temporary camps were replaced by tiny, cramped, permanent dwellings in crowded villages, allowing airborne microbes easy access to their hosts; while food and water, previously collected daily, were now stored in unhygienic conditions, enhancing faecal–oral transmission of gut-infecting microbes. The major factor in introducing new microbes to the early farmers was their close proximity to recently domesticated animals that now shared their dwellings, and which carried their own private microbial zoos.

As we have seen in Chapter 1, the molecular clock technique shows that smallpox virus is most closely related to the pox viruses of camels and gerbils, and not to cowpox as was previously supposed. Scientists think that the rodent pox virus probably jumped to humans and camels in the early farming period, estimating that the event took place some time between 5,000 and 10,000 years ago. In contrast, measles virus's closest relative is Rinderpest virus, the cause of cattle plague, and scientists calculate that the two viruses diverged from a common ancestor around 2,000 years ago. So it seems that these and many other animal microbes infected humans when they first came into close contact during the early farming era. These were the emerging viruses of the period and, as is the way with most emerging infections, at first each epidemic began with transfer of the virus from animal to human host and ended when most susceptible people in the population were infected. Then, as trading links between villages, towns, and countries expanded, these 'new' viruses followed along, causing ever larger and more widespread epidemics.

Studies on measles virus outbreaks in island populations of varying sizes, such as Iceland, Greenland, Fiji, and Hawaii, have been used to estimate the minimum population size required for the virus to circulate continuously in a community, as opposed to it being introduced from outside, at the beginning of each epidemic. The results show that a population of around 500,000 is sufficient, a figure that is probably similar for other airborne viruses. We know that the first towns of this size evolved around 5000 BC in the Fertile Crescent, and so from this time onwards, viruses like measles could break the link with their animal hosts to become entirely human pathogens.

Viruses spread between hosts in many different ways, but those that cause acute epidemics generally utilize fast and efficient methods, such as the airborne or faecal–oral routes. The former is the most efficient method of spread in industrialized nations where people tend to live in crowded towns and cities, whereas this is outstripped by the latter in non-industrialized countries, particularly where standards of hygiene are low.

Broadly speaking, virus infections are distinguished by the organs they affect, with airborne viruses mainly causing respiratory illnesses, like flu, the common cold, or pneumonia, and those transmitted by faecal–oral contamination causing intestinal upsets, with nausea, vomiting, and diarrhoea. There are literally thousands of viruses capable of causing human epidemics, but only a few cause distinctive childhood diseases like measles, mumps, chickenpox, and, until quite recently, smallpox.

Airborne viruses

Smallpox virus is in a class of its own as the world's worst killer virus. We know that it first infected humans at least 5,000 years ago and killed around 300 million in the 20th century alone. The Antonine plague, which began in AD 166, is thought to represent the first ever smallpox pandemic. The plague hit the Roman Empire during the reign of Emperor Marcus Aurelius Antoninus, who ruled over an area encompassing most of modern-day Europe, the Middle East, and North Africa. It began in Seleucia, a city on the River Tigris, while Roman soldiers were suppressing an uprising, and as they returned victorious to Rome, they carried the virus with them, broadcasting it along the way. Over the next 20 years, smallpox raged like a plague throughout the Empire and beyond to India and China, and killed 5,000 a day in Rome at its height. The Romans believed that the plague was punishment meted out by the gods for the sacking of Seleucia, particularly for the opening of a sealed tomb in the temple of Apollo. Marcus Aurelius's physician, Galen of Pergamum, described a 'fever plague' inducing severe thirst, vomiting, and diarrhoea, as well as a rash of fever blisters that were dry, black, and ulcerating – very suggestive of smallpox.

From this time on, smallpox produced ever-increasing epidemics as towns and cities grew and became more crowded. The virus killed up to 30% of those it infected, scarring and blinding many of the survivors. But after centuries of devastation, smallpox virus was finally eliminated from the wild in 1980. The fight to prevent and eliminate smallpox is recounted in Chapter 8.

Until the 1960s, almost every child suffered from the classic childhood virus infections measles, mumps, and rubella, but following the introduction of vaccination programmes these have become a rarity in the developed world. All three viruses access the body through the nose and mouth and colonize the local lymph glands. Then, after a two-week incubation period, during which the victim is blissfully unaware of the invader growing inside them, the viruses travel in the bloodstream to internal organs. This viraemia induces non-specific symptoms like fever, malaise, headache, and runny nose as each virus homes to its particular target organs and the characteristic signs of the illness appear: the tell-tale rashes of measles and rubella, and the painful, swollen parotid glands of mumps. These diseases may be mild in most cases, and recovery leads to lifelong immunity, but each is associated with severe complications that make their prevention worldwide an essential goal.

Of the three viruses, measles is the most infectious and produces the severest disease. It killed millions of children each year before vaccination was introduced in the mid-20th century. Even today, this virus kills over 300,000 children annually in countries with low vaccine coverage. Most deaths from measles result from pneumonia, caused either by the measles virus itself or by other microbes invading the damaged lungs. In developing countries, measles kills 1–5% of those it infects, but this may reach 30% in severely overcrowded living conditions such as refugee camps. The high mortality has long been assumed to be due to pre-existing malnutrition and other debilitating diseases such as malaria, but recent studies in Guinea-Bissau pinpoint another risk factor. They found that measles mortality was higher in rural areas where there are longer intervals between epidemics. This means that rural children experience measles at an older age than urban children. During a rural epidemic, more children per household are susceptible and are often infected sequentially, one from another, in a single epidemic. In this situation, mortality is higher in the second and third child to be infected than in the first (index) case. The reason is that measles virus is mainly spread by droplets generated by coughing, and it is most infectious over short distances in enclosed spaces. Thus, in this study, scientists argued that the index case most probably acquired the virus outside the home, where a low infecting viral dose is likely to result in a relatively mild illness. In contrast, the dose would be higher in the second family member infected from the first because of a cramped and crowded home. And if the more severe the infection, the more virus produced by sequential sufferers, then the dose received would escalate in the family chain along with the disease severity.

Because humans are the only host for measles virus, and the vaccine is safe and highly effective, measles eradication is feasible, and indeed has been achieved in the US, UK, and Australia over prolonged time periods. The Measles Initiative of 2001, set up with the eventual goal of worldwide measles elimination, had already reduced global measles deaths by 74% worldwide by 2005, mostly by increasing vaccine coverage in sub-Saharan Africa and the Eastern Mediterranean and Western Pacific regions. Now the immediate aim is to prevent 90% of measles deaths worldwide and to eradicate the virus by 2020 (see Chapter 8).

Rubella is commonly called German measles because it was first described by a German doctor, Friedrich Hoffmann (1660–1742), in the 18th century, and it was distinguished from measles and scarlet fever by another German doctor, George de Maton, in the 19th century. The infection is generally mild, short-lived, and often passes unnoticed. It would be of little importance if that were the end of the story, but in the 1940s an Australian physician, Norman Gregg (1892–1966), noticed an association between rubella in pregnant mothers and congenital defects in their infants, commonly heart and eye abnormalities and hearing loss. Rubella virus in the mother's blood crosses the placenta and grows in the baby, whose immune system is too immature to respond. This damages the baby's developing organs, and the risk period coincides with organ formation between 10 and 16 weeks of pregnancy. Rubella vaccine is generally given along with measles and mumps vaccines in the MMR vaccine preparation, and has virtually eliminated congenital rubella in countries where vaccine coverage is high, but the condition remains a problem in developing countries.

Mumps is also a relatively mild disease, particularly in childhood, when it may, like rubella, pass unnoticed. Vaccination is advised to prevent the severe complications of meningitis, encephalitis, and orchitis (inflammation of the testis). The latter develops in around 30% of males who catch mumps after puberty and is often bilateral, a condition that may lead to infertility.

Chickenpox is still rife in the UK, and is one of the commonest acute childhood infections worldwide. It rips through children's nurseries and schools on a regular basis, infecting almost all susceptible children before moving on. However, an effective vaccine is available and is given to all children in the US, Canada, Australia, and some European countries, but is not used routinely in the UK. Although chickenpox behaves like a classic acute infectious disease analogous to measles, mumps, and rubella, the virus remains in the body for life after the initial infection and may later resurface to cause shingles. This virus is covered in more detail, along with other persistent viruses, in Chapter 6.

Most people get two or three colds a year, suggesting that the immune system, which is so good at protecting us against a second attack of measles, mumps, or rubella, is defeated by the common cold virus. But this is not the case. In fact, there are so many viruses out there that cause the typical symptoms of blocked nose, headache, malaise, sore throat, sneezing, coughing, and sometimes fever, that even if we live for 100 years, we will not experience them all. The common cold virus, or rhinovirus, alone has over 100 different types, and there are many other viruses that infect the cells lining the nose and throat and cause similar symptoms, often with subtle variations. For example, unlike most respiratory viruses that spread best in the winter months, coxsackie viruses often cause summer colds, and echo- and adenoviruses may produce additional sore red eyes, a condition called conjunctivitis. All these viruses produce local symptoms after two or three days' incubation period that last three to four days and require no treatment. However, infection often leads to loss of work or study time, and because the infections are so common, the global economic burden is enormous.

As any parent knows, young children are very prone to upper respiratory tract infections – the familiar 'snotty-nosed kid'. They are susceptible to the large number of respiratory viruses circulating in the community at any one time, and although most infections are mild, any of these viruses can cause more severe disease, particularly in infants. An infection that spreads to the lower bronchial passages causing bronchiolitis, pneumonia, or croup can be alarming and may require hospital treatment. Viruses

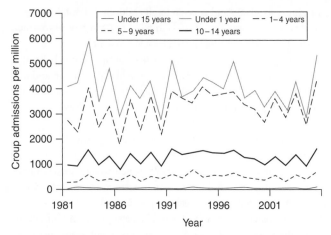

12. Graph showing the number of croup hospitalizations in children under 15 years of age in the USA, 1981 to 2002

such as parainfluenza and respiratory syncytial virus are particularly associated with these problems in infants, regularly causing epidemics and a peak in hospital admissions (Figure 12). Indeed, worldwide acute respiratory infections, mostly viral, cause an estimated four million deaths a year in children under 5.

Anyone who confidently states that they have been off work for a few days with 'the flu' is likely to have suffered from one of the many cold-causing viruses, but a genuine attack of flu caused by influenza A or B virus is quite a different matter. Although producing similar respiratory symptoms, flu has more severe constitutional effects with additional aching muscles and fever, often lasting for seven days. Even after recovery, sufferers may feel lethargic and depressed for a while, further delaying their return to work. In temperate climates, flu A and B outbreaks occur most winters, with significant mortality, mainly from pneumonia, among the very young, very old, and those with other debilitating diseases. Furthermore, the economic burden through loss of work

58

time and hospital admissions is great enough for governments to seek preventive and curative strategies.

Faecal–oral transmission

Viruses that target the gut are just as diverse as respiratory viruses and, in the same way, the hundreds of different gut virus types can attack throughout life. These viruses are spread either directly by unwashed hands or via drinking water, food, and contaminated objects like surfaces and blankets; they are also highly adapted to our bodies and our lifestyle. They survive the acid environment of the stomach that kills most other invaders and then attack the gut lining, killing the cells and thereby stopping the production of digestive enzymes and preventing fluid absorption. All this induces the unpleasant symptoms of gastroenteritis. These viruses manufacture huge numbers of offspring that can survive for long periods outside the body, and infect with a very low virus dose. After an incubation period of between one and two days, the two key culprits, rotaviruses and noroviruses, induce sudden onset of projectile vomiting, profuse watery diarrhoea, and abdominal cramps, which effectively contaminate the environment and ensure their own survival.

Rotaviruses are a major cause of gastroenteritis globally, particularly targeting children under 5. The disease varies in severity but usually lasts four to seven days, with the main problem being dehydration. Indeed, rotaviruses cause over 600,000 infant deaths a year worldwide, mostly in developing countries where the viruses spread easily and emergency rehydration procedures are not always available. With up to a hundred billion (10^{11}) virus particles in each millilitre of faeces produced by an infected child, and only 10 virus particles actually required to pass the infection on, it is not surprising that rotavirus outbreaks are frequent and difficult to control.

As they circulate in the community, rotaviruses, like flu viruses, undergo genetic drift, accumulating point mutations until they are sufficiently different to infect those already immune to the parent virus strain. Also, many strains of rotavirus cause gastroenteritis in young animals such as calves, piglets, lambs, foals, chickens, and rabbits, which can act as rotavirus reservoirs. Again, like flu viruses, from time to time human rotaviruses undergo a genetic shift by gene reassortment with animal rotaviruses. This can produce an entirely new strain with the potential to cause a widespread epidemic.

Noroviruses are the second most common cause of viral gastroenteritis after rotaviruses, producing a milder disease of shorter duration. These viruses account for around 23 million cases of gastroenteritis every year, with epidemics commonly centring on nursing homes, hospitals, and children's nurseries, camps, and schools. Unusually, immunological memory to noroviruses tends to be short, so epidemics affect adults as well as children. Outbreaks among the passengers and staff of cruise ships often hit the headlines, not only ruining the luxury holiday for those on board but also causing severe loss of revenue for the cruise company as ships often have to be taken out of service while the source of the outbreak is identified and the ship disinfected. In a recent example, a cruise ship bound for Alaska set sail from Vancouver with 1,218 passengers and 564 crew on board. The very next day, 5 passengers came down with gastroenteritis, and by the time they disembarked 7 days later, a total of 176 people had reported sick. In port, the ship was disinfected before taking on another group of holidaymakers, this time 1,336 passengers and 571 crew. On this trip, 219 people developed gastroenteritis, necessitating cancellation of the next cruise while the ship was subject to 'aggressive cleaning and sanitizing'. The environmental health inspectors could find no source of infection or 'sanitary deficiencies'. This is commonly the case, and it just goes to show what an effective spreading strategy these viruses have evolved. The virus induces projectile vomiting, a single episode of which releases up to three million virus particles, theoretically enough to infect 300,000 people.

Enteroviruses are an unusual group of viruses because although, as the name suggests, they spread by the faecal–oral route, infect the gut, and are excreted in faeces, they only cause problems if they spread to other organs. Poliovirus is the best known in the group as it can cause a life-threatening disease, paralytic poliomyelitis, but only in around 1 in 1,000 of those it infects.

Like other enteric viruses, poliovirus can survive happily for long periods in water and sewage, so, where standards of hygiene are low, it spreads rapidly among young children. Polioviruses grow in the lining cells of the gut and its associated lymph glands, producing no symptoms but, in a few cases, they target nervous tissues, where they may cause severe disease. In the unlucky few, the virus homes to the brain, causing meningitis (called non-paralytic polio), or to the spinal cord, where it destroys nerve cells and paralyses the related muscles (paralytic polio). The latter is fatal in around 5% of cases, mainly when the paralysis involves the respiratory muscles, leading to respiratory failure.

Poliomyelitis is a disease of modern times, having risen to prominence in the West only in the 20th century. At one time, it caused terrifying summer outbreaks, seeming to strike indiscriminatingly at perfectly healthy children rather than spread from person to person. This was only halted when the vaccine was introduced in the 1960s (see Chapter 8). In developing countries at this time and, it is assumed, before the 20th century in industrialized countries, polioviruses circulated freely in the community and infected virtually the whole population during early childhood. In this situation, paralytic poliomyelitis was almost unknown. The silent nature of the infection is thought to result from residual maternal antibodies which passed across the placenta while the child was *in utero* and protected it from paralytic disease by preventing viral spread outside the gut. Then, as standards of hygiene rose and infection in infancy became less common, many mothers remained uninfected and so had not generated antibodies that could be passed on to, and protect, their infants. Thus the incidence of paralytic polio was inversely related to levels of hygiene, rising along with industrialization of a nation.

Many virus families such as rotaviruses that rely on faecal–oral transmission and cause gastroenteritis in humans produce the same symptoms in animals, resulting in great economic loss to the farming industry. However, over the centuries, Rinderpest virus, the cause of cattle plague, has probably been responsible for more loss and hardship than any other. Rinderpest virus is closely related to measles virus, but the disease it causes is very different. The virus infects cloven-hoofed animals such as oxen, buffalo, yak, sheep, goats, pigs, camels, and several wild species including hippopotamus, giraffe, and warthog. It usually spreads by direct contact, entering via the mouth, growing in lymph glands of the nose and throat, and producing a nasal discharge. From here, the infection extends to the whole length of the gut, causing severe ulceration. Rinderpest is classically described by the three Ds: discharge, diarrhoea, and death, the latter being caused by fluid loss with rapid dehydration. The disease kills around 90% of animals infected.

Rinderpest used to be a major problem in Europe and Asia, and when it was introduced into Africa in the late 19th century, it killed over 90% of cattle, with devastating economic loss. The Global Rinderpest Eradication Programme was set up in the 1980s aiming to use the effective vaccine to rid the world of the virus by 2010. This was successful, and in October 2010 the disease was officially declared eradicated, the first animal disease and second infectious disease ever to be eliminated.

Many acute infectious viruses thrive in hospital and care home settings, causing outbreaks of hospital-acquired, or nosocomial, infections. Although today's headlines are generally dominated by notorious bacterial infections like MRSA (methicillin-resistant *Staphylococcus aureus*), *Clostridium difficile*, and the 'flesh-eating bug' *Streptococcus pyogenes*, nosocomial virus infections go unreported and are in fact a common cause of outbreaks severe enough to lead to ward closures.

Unfortunately, in the close confines of a hospital ward, patients are easy prey for viruses. Viruses that circulate in the community causing silent or mild infections can be devastating to premature babies, those debilitated by cancer or other chronic illnesses, the elderly, and the immunosuppressed. Most often, a recently admitted patient is the source of the infection but, not uncommonly, it is a staff member who may remain healthy and be totally unaware that he or she is spreading a potentially lethal virus. Norovirus, with its abrupt onset of projectile vomiting, is particularly difficult to control and, because its incubation period of 1 to 2 days is too short to allow identification of the source in time to prevent secondary spread, it is often the reason for ward closures.

In some outbreaks, hospitals may even be responsible for amplifying an infection, with spread to the community outside the hospital before the problem is recognized. This clearly happened with SARS in Hong Kong when a hospital visitor carried the virus to Amoy Gardens, a private housing estate, where it infected over 300 people, of whom 42 died. Also, before an outbreak of Ebola virus is recognized as such, the infection is often carried from a hospitalized patient via staff or visitors out into the community.

Interestingly, in recent years measles has become a problem in the hospital setting. Because of the rarity of measles in countries with high vaccine coverage, cases often go undiagnosed until the rash appears, by which time the patient has been infectious for several days. These days, most measles index cases in hospitals are imported, mainly by unvaccinated staff or patients who come from, or have recently visited, countries where vaccine coverage is poor.

Strict barrier nursing must be implemented immediately to prevent spread to those with weakened immune systems, among whom mortality from measles can reach 50%.

The growing problem of hospital-acquired infections now requires teams of experts in infection control in every hospital to block their transmission. In the next chapter, we look at virus infections that cannot be prevented in this way as they are carried by an individual for life, taking advantage of any dip in immunity to replicate in their host and thereby spread to others.

Chapter 6
Persistent viruses

Viruses fight a constant battle against host immunity, and for most there is just a small window of opportunity in which to reproduce and make a hasty exit before being wiped out by the formidable array of host defences. But some viruses have evolved strategies for overcoming these immune mechanisms and survive inside their host for prolonged periods, even for a lifetime. Although the detailed mechanisms involved in these evasion strategies are very complex and varied, overall they encompass three basic manoeuvres: finding a niche in which to hide from immune attack, manipulating immune processes to benefit the virus, and outwitting immune defences by mutating rapidly.

Most persistent viruses have evolved to cause mild or even asymptomatic infections, since a life-threatening disease would not only be detrimental to the host but also deprive the virus of its home. Indeed, some viruses apparently cause no ill effects at all, and have been discovered only by chance. One example is TTV, a tiny DNA virus found in 1997 during the search for the cause of hepatitis and named after the initials (TT) of the patient from whom it was first isolated. We now know that TTV, and its relative TTV-like mini virus, represent a whole spectrum of similar viruses that are carried by almost all humans, non-human primates, and a variety of other vertebrates, but so far they have not been associated with any disease. With modern, highly sensitive molecular techniques for identifying non-pathogenic viruses, we can expect to find more of these silent passengers in the future.

The frequency with which viruses succeed in persisting in their hosts varies, with herpesviruses virtually always establishing a lifelong relationship that usually does no harm to the host. Retroviruses also generally infect for life, but they may, like HIV, cause a disease in those they infect after a prolonged silent period. Other viruses, such as hepatitis B virus, struggle to evade the immune response, and many hosts eventually manage to clear the virus. Further, there are a few viruses that are usually cleared after primary infection but on rare occasions may stay put. Measles virus, for example, for unknown reasons persists after the acute infection in around 1 in 10,000 cases causing a fatal brain disease called subacute sclerosing pan encephalitis (SSPE).

Because of the lifelong presence of foreign (viral) genes inside a host cell, a persistent virus can sometimes drive the cell it lodges in into uncontrolled growth, that is, to become cancerous. These include human T lymphotropic virus, hepatitis B and C viruses, Epstein–Barr virus, Kaposi sarcoma-associated virus, and the papilloma viruses. The mechanisms involved in the evolution of these cancers are dealt with in Chapter 7.

The herpesvirus family

Herpesviruses form an ancient family whose common ancestor probably evolved during the Devonian period around 400 million years ago when fish-like creatures were just emerging from the seas to inhabit dry land. In doing so, they must have encountered an array of 'new' microbes, among them the primitive phage-like viruses thought to be the ancestors of modern-day herpesviruses.

From this early beginning, herpesviruses have co-evolved with their hosts, each partner exerting selective pressure on the other until they have become remarkably well adapted to each other's lifestyles, allowing the viruses to thrive long term, generally without detriment to the hosts. As their host species diverged, herpesviruses also diverged, so that now almost all species of mammals, birds, reptiles, amphibians, fish, and even some non-vertebrates, have their own particular herpesvirus cocktail.

To date, over 150 different herpesviruses have been identified, all of which are large, enveloped DNA viruses coding for between 80 and 150 proteins. They are fragile viruses that cannot survive independently for long in the outside world, and so they tend to spread by close contact between infectious and susceptible hosts.

Without exception, herpesviruses establish a lifelong infection, often called a *latent infection*. The viruses survive inside host cells in a dormant state, having shut down their protein production and thereby having become invisible to host immunity. Occasionally, during the lifetime of the host this latent infection reactivates to produce new viruses. The evolution of this long-term strategy ensures that virus offspring reach a young and susceptible host population and thereby guarantees their survival.

There are three herpesvirus subfamilies: alpha, beta, and gamma, with members categorized according to their biological properties, particularly the cell types in which they establish latency. So far, eight human herpesviruses have been discovered, named herpesvirus (HHV) 1 to 8 in order of their discovery, but also given 'common' names by which they are more familiarly known (see the table).

We inherited these viruses from our primate ancestors, and so each has a counterpart in primates to which it is more closely related than it is to the other human herpesviruses. Having co-evolved with us, herpesviruses infect all human populations worldwide, including the most isolated Amerindian tribes.

Name	Common name	Subfamily	Common primary clinical symptoms	Overall adult prevalence *(%)	Site of latency
HHV-1	Herpes simplex type 1 (HSV-1)	Alpha	Cold sore	>60	Nerve ganglia
HHV-2	Herpes simplex type 2 (HSV-2)	Alpha	Genital herpes	20	Nerve ganglia
HHV-3	Varicella zoster virus (VZV)	Alpha	Chickenpox	~90	Nerve ganglia
HHV-4	Epstein–Barr virus (EBV)	Gamma	Glandular fever	~90	B lymphocytes
HHV-5	Cytomegalovirus (CMV)	Beta	Mononucleosis syndrome	~50	Bone marrow stem cells
HHV-6	–	Beta	Exanthem Subitum	~90	White blood cells
HHV-7	–	Beta	Exanthem Subitum	~90	White blood cells
HHV-8	Kaposi sarcoma-associated herpesvirus (KSHV)	Gamma	–	<5	B lymphocytes

It is generally assumed that in the past all the human herpesviruses were ubiquitous, but today their prevalence varies, the hierarchy perhaps reflecting their success at spreading between hosts in the modern world. Human herpesviruses can spread in a variety of ways: transmitted directly from mother to child in breast milk (CMV) or spread among family members and close contacts via saliva (HSV-1, CMV, EBV, HHV-6 and -7, KSHV). Of these viruses, HHV-6 and -7 are the most successful, infecting almost everyone worldwide. The prevalence of EBV, HSV-1, and CMV is also high, but each has experienced a recent drop in areas where high standards of hygiene tend to block their transmission. Interestingly, HSV-2 and KSHV have a much lower prevalence than the other human herpesviruses and show a more restricted geographical distribution, being most common in parts of Africa. These viruses rely on salivary transmission in childhood (KSHV) and/or sexual transmission between adults, and scientists speculate that they are the most vulnerable to recent cultural and lifestyle changes and therefore their worldwide distribution is the first to be significantly eroded.

The alpha human herpesviruses, HSV-1 and -2, are 85% identical at the DNA level, but traditionally HSV-1 causes a cold sore on the face whereas HSV-2 causes genital herpes. Although this is still generally true, in fact both viruses can infect the skin of the face and genital area, and a rising minority of genital herpes cases are now caused by HSV-1.

HSV-1 and -2 access the body through a cut or abrasion and target skin cells where they replicate, killing the infected cells as new viruses are produced. The majority of primary HSV infections are silent, but they sometimes cause a painful rash of tiny blisters in and around the mouth or in the genital area. With each blister containing thousands of virus particles, it is easy to see how the virus spreads to other individuals.

HSV infection of the skin soon attracts the attention of immune cells and the lesions heal rapidly, but not before some virus particles have secretly infected nerve endings in the skin and climbed up the nerve fibres to the cell nucleus where they establish latency. HSV from a facial infection (mainly HSV-1) goes latent in the trigeminal ganglia at the base of the skull, whereas viruses from genital lesions (mainly HSV-2) head for the sacral ganglia alongside the lower spinal column. As nerve cells survive for the life of the host and do not divide, they are an ideal site for a virus to lie low for a while. But to assure its long-term survival, at some stage the virus must wake up and move on. So from time to time, new viruses are produced, which travel down the nerve fibres and are shed into saliva or genital secretions. This reactivation may be silent or may manifest as a cold sore on the face, classically on or near the lips, in around 40% of those carrying HSV-1, and as genital herpes in around 60% of those carrying HSV-2. The triggers for HSV reactivation in an individual carrier are often quite clear and recognizable: decreased immunity due to drugs or illness, fever, increased levels of ultraviolet light (classically precipitated by a skiing trip), or menstruation and stress, but the molecular mechanisms involved are not understood.

Chickenpox, as a very common, acute infection of childhood, has been dealt with in Chapter 5, but being a herpesvirus, VZV establishes a latent infection in virtually everyone it infects. Like the HSVs, VZV hides in nerve cells, but as the chickenpox rash is widespread on the body, the virus may lodge in the spinal ganglia related to any or all of the nerves supplying the skin.

Latent VZV can reactivate to cause shingles at any time in life, but this is most common in the elderly. Reactivation usually occurs in a single nerve cell, causing the typical painful shingles rash of tiny blisters along the course of that particular nerve. As infectious viruses are shed from these lesions, individuals who have not had it before can catch chickenpox from them. But shingles is not caught either from cases of shingles or chickenpox, as it is the result of reactivation of internal, latent viruses.

As with the HSVs, the molecular mechanisms involved in VZV reactivation are unknown, and why it should occur most commonly in nerves supplying the eye, neck, and trunk is also a mystery. However, again similar to HSV, reactivation is more common in patients with immunosuppression, including those who are HIV positive, have had an organ transplant, or are receiving chemotherapy. In all these groups, the rash may be severe, widespread, and even life-threatening, but several antiviral agents, including aciclovir, can have a beneficial effect (see Chapter 8).

Of the three human beta herpesviruses, CMV is the only one that causes significant health problems. Although the virus infects most people silently, it occasionally causes a glandular-fever-like illness at primary infection. But more importantly, the virus in a pregnant woman's blood may on rare occasions cross the placenta and infect her unborn child. When this happens, it causes cytomegalic inclusion disease in around 10% of affected infants, inducing a wide range of symptoms including growth retardation, deafness, abnormalities of blood clotting, and inflammation of the liver, lungs, heart, and brain.

CMV establishes latency in the bone marrow stem cells that develop into blood monocytes and tissue macrophages. These cells transport the latent virus via the blood to the tissues where virus reactivation is common. In healthy hosts, this is dealt with by the immune system without causing disease, but CMV replication produces significant pathology in immunosuppressed patients, and was responsible for blindness, severe diarrhoea, pneumonia, and encephalitis in many HIV-positive people before effective antivirals were developed in the early 1990s.

The two human gamma herpesviruses, EBV and KSHV, are both tumour viruses and as such are dealt with in Chapter 8. However, although KSHV appears to cause no problems on primary infection, EBV may cause glandular fever, also called infectious mononucleosis.

EBV generally infects silently during childhood, but if infection is delayed until adolescence or early adulthood, it causes glandular fever in around one-quarter of cases. As childhood infection is virtually ubiquitous in developing countries, and is also very common in low socioeconomic groups in developed countries, glandular fever is most prevalent in high socioeconomic groups in the developed world. In these situations, it is quite common among senior school pupils and university students, estimated to affect around 1 in 1,000 university students per year in one UK study.

EBV infects and establishes latency in blood B cells, and perhaps because these cells are themselves part of the immune system, the infection engenders an exaggerated T cell response. Indeed, the symptoms of glandular fever, which typically include sore throat, fever, enlarged glands in the neck, and fatigue, are immunopathological in nature, caused by this massive outpouring of T cells rather than directly by the virus infection itself. Although the illness usually resolves over 10 to 14 days, fatigue may persist for up to 6 months, sometimes causing quite severe disruption to the sufferer's way of life.

On rare occasions, EBV causes tumours (see Chapter 8) and has also been suggested as the cause of several other diseases, particularly autoimmune diseases such as rheumatoid arthritis and multiple sclerosis (see Chapter 9).

The retrovirus family

Retroviruses infect a wide range of animal species, often acting as a silent passenger, but sometimes causing immunodeficiency, leukaemia, or solid tumours. There are several retroviruses that cause immunodeficiency in humans all of which have been acquired from primates. Today, these HIVs are the only non-tumour-forming retroviruses to cause disease in humans, but there are intriguing clues to suggest that ancient hominids may have been prey to several more. Evidence for this theory comes from the large number of identifiable retroviral remnants within the human genome, but how and when they got there, and why they have been retained, remains a mystery. Perhaps our ancestors survived the onslaught of these infections by developing resistance while those who did not simply died out.

Human HIVs include not only HIV-1 group M, the pandemic strain of HIV, but also HIV-1 strains N, O, and P, and HIV-2. We now know that all these viruses recently jumped from primates to humans in Africa, and it is probable that such transfers have occurred from time to time throughout our history, but remained unnoticed because they did not spread beyond the immediate area. It was the unique occurrence of HIV-1 group M spread from Africa to Haiti and on to the USA in the 1960s that prompted the first description of AIDS in 1980 and the isolation of the virus in 1983.

HIV-2, discovered in 1986, is only 40% identical to HIV-1 and has a quite distinct origin, having been acquired from the sooty mangabey monkey in West Africa. Although this virus spreads in the same way, infects the same cell types as HIV-1, and also causes AIDS, it is less infectious than HIV-1 and has remained local to West Africa.

HIV-1 and AIDS

Since humans have acquired HIV-1 only recently, we lack genetic resistance to the virus, and thus virtually every untreated infection eventually ends in death from AIDS. Just a few fortunate individuals are resistant to infection, and the mechanism for this is discussed in Chapter 3. Other aspects of HIV-1 have also been discussed earlier: retrovirus biology and HIV receptor usage in Chapter 1, and HIV origin from chimps, its time of transfer to humans, subsequent spread, and eventual discovery in Chapter 4. In this chapter, we concentrate on the consequences of HIV-1 infection and the pathogenesis of AIDS.

Although AIDS was first described in gay men, and shortly afterwards injecting drug users and haemophiliacs were found to be at risk, worldwide the virus is mainly transmitted by heterosexual intercourse. There are now 33 million people living with HIV, with around 2.7 million new infections, and 2 million deaths, per year. The virus has invaded virtually every country in the world, with the overwhelming impact in developing countries; 22 million people are living with HIV in sub-Saharan Africa. But even these startling figures belie the tragedy of the worst-hit African countries where life expectancy has tumbled to below 40 years by the wholesale death of previously healthy and productive adults, creating an economic downturn, severe poverty, and around 15 million AIDS orphans.

HIV infects cells bearing the CD4 marker, mainly helper T cells and tissue macrophages. Virus infection occurs through contact with the blood or genital secretions of a carrier, usually via a tear or abrasion in the epithelium lining the genital tract, or, commonly, an open sore caused by another sexually transmitted infection such as HSV, gonococcus, or syphilis. On entry, the virus initially targets Langerhans cells, the subset of macrophages that patrol the skin and epithelial surfaces, including the lining of the genital tract. These cells then carry the virus to the local lymph glands, where literally millions of CD4 T cells congregate while taking a rest from circulating in the blood. Infection of these long-lived cells not only disseminates the virus throughout the body but also provides a site of persistence as the proviral genome integrates into their DNA.

The clinical course of HIV infection naturally divides into three stages: the acute, the asymptomatic, and the symptomatic phases,

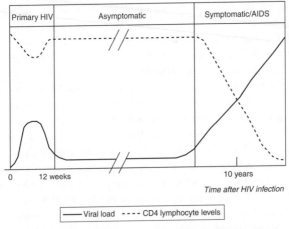

| Primary HIV | Asymptomatic | Symptomatic/AIDS |

| 0 | 12 weeks | 10 years |

Time after HIV infection

——— Viral load - - - - CD4 lymphocyte levels

13. Graph showing the CD4 count and viral load during the acute, asymptomatic, and symptomatic phases of HIV infection

the last being manifest as AIDS (Figure 13). People infected with HIV often experience a primary illness known as the acute retroviral syndrome between one and six weeks after infection. This is a fairly non-specific illness with fever, sore throat, swollen glands, a rash, and general aches and pains, and usually lasts up to 14 days followed by complete recovery.

Initially, the virus multiplies freely in CD4 T cells, destroying over 30 million of them every day. Levels of virus in the blood (called the viral load) rise to a peak in the first few weeks, after which the immune response kicks in, controlling but not completely clearing the virus. The viral load then falls, and by six months it has generally stabilized to a 'set point' level, the height of which depends on the strength of the immune response and is all important in predicting the further course of the disease; the higher the set point, the quicker the progression to AIDS.

In an untreated person, the asymptomatic phase of HIV infection lasts between 6 and 15 years depending on the viral set point, and although carriers in this phase are generally well, HIV continues its battle with their immune system, causing cumulative damage. Early on, the HIV genome in infected cells is fairly uniform, but the more it replicates, the more it throws up mutants, some of which can evade the immune response. As these mutants prosper, an arms race develops between immune T cells and antibodies, on the one hand, and a series of immunity-evading virus mutants, on the other. CD4 T cells are pivotal to the continually evolving immune response, but HIV replicates in these cells and destroys them at such a rate that the body cannot keep pace. Eventually, the CD4 cell production line runs dry and numbers decline. Without antiviral drugs to control virus replication, the body's capacity to replenish CD4 cells is eventually exhausted, such that when the level drops below the critical threshold of 200 CD4 cells per millilitre of blood, immunity to other pathogens fails and they take the opportunity to invade.

Evidence of declining immunity and the imminent onset of the symptomatic phase of the HIV infection, AIDS, often includes weight loss, night sweats, recurrent chest infections, skin lesions such as warts, and oral ulcers and infections like thrush and cold sores. These are then followed by the relentless onslaught of a plethora of opportunistic infections, including reactivation of persistent microbes like CMV, HSV, VZV, and TB, as well as tumours caused by HPV, KSHV, and EBV. One of the hallmarks of AIDS is infection with microbes that are no problem to people with healthy immune systems, for example pneumonia caused by avian TB or the fungus *Pneumocystic jirovecii* (previously *P. carinii*) – the latter provided the clue to the recognition of AIDS as a new disease in 1980.

Central nervous system manifestations are also common in AIDS, as HIV invades the brain at an early stage of the disease, infecting and killing cells, causing progressive degenerative changes leading to AIDS-associated encephalopathy and dementia. In addition, CMV and another very common, persistent, and generally asymptomatic virus called JC (from the initials of the patient from whom it was first isolated) may cause progressive degenerative brain disease in AIDS sufferers.

Death from one of these infections inevitably follows, often within months. Fortunately, today antiretroviral therapy has transformed this grim picture of HIV infection into a treatable chronic disease, but this treatment is not without its problems, and there are still millions of HIV sufferers in the developing world who have no access to these life-saving drugs which are discussed in Chapter 8.

Hepatitis viruses

Hepatitis, meaning inflammation of the liver, can be caused by a variety of viruses as well as toxic chemicals such as alcohol and the drug paracetamol. The liver is a huge organ with plenty of spare capacity, so mild inflammation often passes unnoticed. The main indication of more severe damage is the yellow discolouration of the skin known as jaundice, often most noticeable in the whites of the eyes.

Several viruses, including Epstein–Barr and herpes simplex viruses, can cause hepatitis as part of a generalized infection, but for others the liver is their main site of replication, causing them to be lumped together as 'the hepatitis viruses' although they belong to quite different virus families. To date, five human hepatitis viruses have been discovered and named A, B, C, D, and E. With the exception of HDV, all these viruses either infect silently or produce clinical hepatitis varying in severity from mild and self-limiting to fulminant – that is, acute liver failure which is generally fatal unless a liver transplant can be performed as an emergency procedure.

Hepatitis A and E viruses spread by the faecal–oral route causing epidemics of 'infectious jaundice', and where standards of hygiene are low most children are infected at an early age. Although the illness may be prolonged, recovery is the rule, and the viruses do not persist thereafter. In contrast, hepatitis B and C viruses may persist after primary infection, and this can lead to chronic hepatitis, cirrhosis, and liver cancer. Hepatitis D virus (HDV), also known as delta virus, is unique among human viruses in being defective and requiring the assistance of HBV for its transmission. Specifically, HDV particles consist of an RNA genome surrounded by their own protein but enveloped in HBV surface antigen that acts as its receptor for getting in and out of liver cells. So this virus can only replicate in cells already infected with HBV and manufacturing HBV surface antigen. HDV may be transmitted along with HBV or may infect an HBV carrier, and in both cases it tends to worsen the infection by increasing the liver damage and accelerating the onset of chronic liver disease.

Hepatitis C virus is mainly spread by blood contamination. Once routine testing of donor blood excluded most HBV-infected units in the 1970s, HCV became the commonest cause of viral hepatitis following blood transfusion. But after its discovery in 1989, when blood and blood products were screened for HCV, the commonest route of transmission became needle sharing by intravenous drug users. Around 10% of carrier mothers pass the virus to their newborn offspring, but household and sexual contacts are not thought to be at increased risk.

HCV presently infects around 170 million people. Infection occurs worldwide but shows marked geographical variation, with 1–2% of the population infected in the USA, northern Europe, and Australia, and rates of up to 5% in southern and central Europe, Japan, and parts of the Middle East (Figure 14). The highest levels of around 20% are recorded in Egypt, where a treatment programme for the parasitic disease bilharzia in the 1960s unwittingly spread the virus by using non-sterile needles.

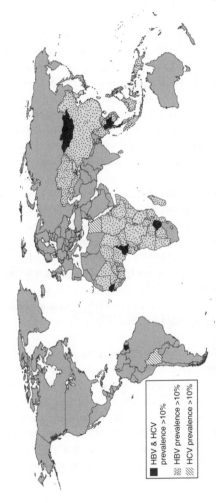

HBV & HCV
prevalence >10%

HBV prevalence >10%

HCV prevalence >10%

14. World map showing the prevalence of HBV and HCV infections

Only about one-quarter of those with primary HCV infection develop hepatitis with symptoms, but whether symptomatic or not, around 80% of acute HCV cases progress to a chronic phase.

HCV has many ways of dodging the body's immunity. As an RNA virus, HCV, like HIV, mutates rapidly and this, combined with its extremely high replication rate, generates a whole array of minor genetic variants, called quasispecies, in a single individual. Some of these variants manage to evade immune T cells and antibodies generated specifically to combat the virus, and these mutants then flourish until the immune response catches up with them. Then another viral variant will come to prominence, and this immune-driven evolution will continue to foil host immunity *ad infinitum*.

HCV also evades host immunity by blocking antiviral mechanisms inside infected cells, preventing the production of cytokines like interferon that might otherwise curtail its spread in the liver. The virus also induces regulatory T cells that paradoxically damp down anti-HCV immunity. The importance of this is demonstrated by the finding that during primary HCV, the height of this response reflects the outcome: those with a high level of regulatory T cells have a higher viral load and are more likely to develop a persistent infection than those with a lower level of the same cells.

It is not clear whether the liver damage caused by HCV infection is directly due to virus replication in liver cells or to immunopathology, but whatever the mechanism, there are signs of ongoing liver damage in all chronic HCV carriers, many of whom are unaware of the infection, and this progresses to chronic active hepatitis and/or cirrhosis in up to 70% of cases. Intensive antiviral treatment can clear the virus in some cases, but this is expensive and only affordable by health services in the developed world (see Chapter 8).

No vaccine is available to prevent HCV infection, and with 3% of the world's population currently infected, this is now the commonest cause of liver failure and indication for liver transplantation in the Western world. Chronic HCV infection is also associated with the development of liver cancer (see Chapter 7), and in countries where HBV prevalence has decreased due to the screening of donor blood and more recent vaccination programmes, HCV is now the major risk factor for this tumour.

HBV was discovered by chance in 1964 in the blood of an Australian Aborigine and shown to be a major cause of transfusion-associated hepatitis. The virus is extremely infectious and carriers have high viral loads in blood and body fluids. It spreads by close contact, particularly sexual intercourse, and mother to child, as well as by blood contamination of medical instruments, dental drills, and needles used for injection, and household utensils such as razors, toothbrushes, and by tattooing, body piercing, and acupuncture. Intravenous drug users and gay men are at particular risk of infection.

Around 350 million people worldwide carry HBV, with many more showing evidence of past infection. The prevalence varies geographically with South-East Asia and sub-Saharan Africa having the highest levels (Figure 14).

Like the other hepatitis virus infections, primary HBV infection is usually silent, and most healthy adults clear the virus within six months. Just 1–5% of adult cases lead to lifelong persistence, and this may cause liver damage, cirrhosis, and/or cancer later in life. Most persistent infections are the result of infection early in life, particularly when the virus is passed from a viraemic mother to her child at the time of birth. Due to the immaturity of the immune system, over 90% of these perinatal cases develop persistence unless they receive prompt treatment at birth. With over 10 million DNA copies per millilitre of blood, spread to other children is a common occurrence.

Levels of HBV infection dropped following screening of blood and blood products, and the vaccine that was introduced in 1982 has succeeded in breaking the cycle of mother to child spread in countries where this was the major route of transmission. However, HBV is still a large problem worldwide because many carriers do not know that they are infected until they develop fatal consequences. Now that there are effective ways to control the infection with antiviral drugs (see Chapter 8), there is a case for screening all those in risk groups. This would allow the early identification and treatment of carriers and prevention by vaccination in those found to be uninfected.

Persistent viruses are well-adapted parasites whose lifestyle is intricately balanced to their host. Most maintain a benign presence for the lifetime of the host, but in a few cases the balance is upset and disease, including cancer, ensues. In the next chapter, we examine the mechanisms behind virus-associated cancer development.

Chapter 7
Tumour viruses

The history of tumour virology began in 1908 when two Danish scientists, Wilhelm Ellermann and Oluf Bang, transmitted chicken leukaemia from a leukaemic bird to a healthy bird by injection of a filtered extract of leukaemic cells. The importance of this experiment was not fully appreciated at the time as leukaemia was not generally recognized as a malignant disease, and it was only after US scientist Peyton Rous transmitted a solid tumour from tumour-bearing to healthy chickens in 1911 that the findings had an impact. Both experiments indicated that some kind of 'filterable agent' was involved in tumour development, yet they pre-dated the identification and characterization of viruses. Due to this lack of knowledge and the fact that tumours do not generally behave like an infectious disease, the scientific community was slow to grasp their importance. Indeed, Rous had to wait over 50 years before he was awarded a Nobel Prize for his work on what became known as the 'Rous sarcoma virus'.

Over the intervening years, other pioneering tumour virologists began to uncover the complex molecular mechanisms involved in tumour development. Using a combination of tumour-susceptible strains of laboratory animals and cell culture techniques, they identified specific viral genes which could convert, or transform, normal cells into tumour-like cells in a culture dish and also induce them to form tumours in laboratory animals. These genes are called viral oncogenes, and unravelling the various ways in which they transform cells has been instrumental in uncovering the molecular mechanisms involved in cancer development in general. Most importantly, the discovery in the 1980s that viral oncogenes have counterparts in the normal cellular genome (called proto-oncogenes) led to the realization that some time in the distant past these tumour viruses must have picked up, or transduced, their oncogenes from the cells they infect.

Tumours develop when a single cell in an organism is somehow released from the usual constraints that regulate its growth, and it replicates unchecked. This rogue cell then produces a mass of similar cells, forming a tumour (or cancer) that invades the surrounding tissues and may spread from its original site.

Healthy cells are subject to many complex chemical checks and balances which ensure that they grow and divide, age and die, only when appropriate. Not surprisingly, therefore, the development of a cancer cell involves mutations that alter the function of the genes that regulate these vital cellular controls. Both an increase in the action of genes that drive cell proliferation (called cellular oncogenes and including the proto-oncogenes that some tumour viruses have picked up) and a decrease in function of genes that inhibit cell division or induce cell death (called tumour suppressor genes) will have the effect of releasing the cell from normal constraints in favour of uncontrolled proliferation.

One in three people develop cancer at some time during their lives, resulting in nearly 11 million new cases, and well over 6 million deaths worldwide every year. For most, the cause is unknown, although there are some well-known associations with environmental factors. Common examples are smoking that predisposes to lung cancer, exposure to strong sunlight that is linked to skin cancer, and asbestos inhalation that causes a tumour of the cells lining the lungs called a mesothelioma. However, the onset of cancer is not an abrupt process resulting from a single cellular event, but a long journey during which the cell undergoes a series of 'hits' that induce mutations and eventually turn it into a cancer cell. One of these hits could be exposure to tobacco, UV irradiation, or asbestos. Now that the whole human genome has been sequenced, scientists have catalogued the mutations in cancer cells and have found that there are literally thousands. One of the cancer-inducing cellular hits may be infection with a virus, but since many more hits are required to produce a cancer cell, a tumour is usually a rare and late outcome of infection with a tumour virus.

Human tumour viruses

After the link between viruses and tumours in animals was finally accepted, scientists still struggled to find similar associations in humans, and many began to doubt their existence. Even when the first candidate human tumour viruses were finally identified in the 1960s, general acceptance was slow in coming. Again, there was no obvious sign that they were infectious, and the virus infection turned out to be far more common and widespread than the tumours they were supposed to cause. Many believed that the associations were chance findings and viruses were just 'passengers' in the tumour cells rather than driving their growth. Indeed, it is still very difficult to provide watertight proof of a viral cause for a human cancer, or even draw up criteria that must be met to substantiate the association, as each virus uses different mechanisms and tumour development often involves co-factors with their own particular characteristics. However, in general, the following criteria should apply:

- The geographical distribution of the virus coincides with that of the tumour;
- The incidence of the virus infection is higher in tumour-bearing than healthy subjects;

- Virus infection precedes tumour development;
- Tumour incidence is decreased by prevention of the virus infection;
- Tumour incidence is increased in immunocompromised people.

For a suspected tumour virus:

- The viral genome is present in tumour but not in normal cells;
- The virus can transform cells in a culture system;
- The virus can induce tumours in experimental animals.

Worldwide, 10–20% of human cancers are linked to viruses, including some common tumours like cervical cancer in women and liver cancer, which is more common in men. So far, all the human tumour viruses discovered are persistent viruses that successfully evade their hosts' immune attack and remain on board long term. This is a rather comfortable position for a virus to be in, and it is hard to see why it should evolve tumorigenic properties since killing its host is not advantageous to its survival. But now that the mechanisms involved in viral oncogenesis are at least partially understood, it is clear that cell transformation generally results from the misuse of functions vital for the virus's survival and that it generally involves a number of co-factors. The exceptions to this rule are oncogenic members of the retrovirus family that carry oncogenes that act directly to transform a cell.

Oncogenic retroviruses

Although most human tumour viruses known today are persistent DNA viruses, the first animal tumour viruses to be discovered, including Rous sarcoma virus, were mostly RNA retroviruses. Uniquely, when these viruses infect a cell, they produce a DNA copy of their RNA genome, a provirus, which inserts into the cellular genome and thereafter is replicated along with cellular DNA (see Chapter 1). This remarkable feat not only protects the virus from immune attack and ensures its survival for the lifetime of the cell, but also has the potential to reprogramme the cell's own gene expression, so influencing its growth control mechanisms.

The only human oncogenic retrovirus identified to date is human T lymphotropic virus that belongs to a group of large retroviruses which also includes the simian and bovine leukaemia viruses. These three viruses do not contain genes transduced from their hosts but have a region in the genome called pX containing genes with a variety of functions including cell transformation. However, all three viruses only rarely cause tumours, and then only many years after the initial infection. This suggests that the infection is not enough on its own and some as yet unknown cellular mutations must be instrumental in tumour progression.

Human T lymphotropic virus (HTLV-1)

HTLV-1 infects approximately 20 million people in distinct geographical areas around the world. Fortunately, only a small percentage of these carriers develop HTLV-1-related diseases, generally after a latent period lasting for several decades. These diseases include adult T cell leukaemia and the non-malignant myelopathy, also called tropical spastic paraparesis. The latter is a chronic neurological illness that causes progressive disability over decades, with over half the sufferers eventually becoming immobile.

HTLV-1 was first isolated in 1980 by Robert Gallo and his team in Baltimore, USA, during an intensive hunt for human tumour retroviruses. These scientists used the recently identified T cell growth factor called interleukin-2 to grow leukaemic T cells for the first time in culture and combined with new assays for reverse transcriptase (RT), the enzyme produced by replicating retroviruses. They found a culture from just one patient's leukaemic cells that produced RT and eventually isolated HTLV-1 from this patient's cells. Several years earlier, Kiyoshi Takatsuki and colleagues in Kumamoto, Japan, had described a newly recognized disease called adult T cell leukaemia (ATL) with cases particularly clustering in the southwest of the country, a fact that suggested an environmental or infectious cause. In 1981, these scientists isolated a retrovirus from cultured ATL cells which turned out to be identical to HTLV-1.

In addition to Japan, where around 1.2 million people are infected with HTLV-1, the incidence reaching up to 15% in the southwest region, other HTLV-1 high-incidence areas include sub-Saharan Africa, the Caribbean, and some pockets in South America, the Middle East, and Melanesia (see Figure 15). Exactly how the virus reached these disparate populations is not known. Recent molecular studies show that HTLV-1's closest relatives are among the simian retroviruses carried by several Old World monkey species in Africa and Asia, and find evidence of several past transmissions from these animals to humans. Those viruses that thrived in their new host were disseminated by ancient human migrations. One strain is thought to have reached Japan some time before 300 BC, when an invasion from mainland Asia drove the indigenous population to the north and southwest. These are the areas where the highest incidences are found today. Another strain originating in Africa was probably carried to the Caribbean by the slave trade, and from thence to South America.

HTLV-1 primarily infects blood T cells and has three main routes of spread: from mother to child, through sexual intercourse, and by blood contact, including transfusion of blood and cellular blood products and needle sharing among intravenous drug users. In Japan, mother to child transmission is the most common route, mainly via breast feeding, when 25% of the babies of virus-carrying mothers become infected.

HTLV-1 persists in blood T cells for life, but the infection is generally harmless. However, between 2% and 6% of cases progress to ATL or lymphoma, both of which are generally aggressive,

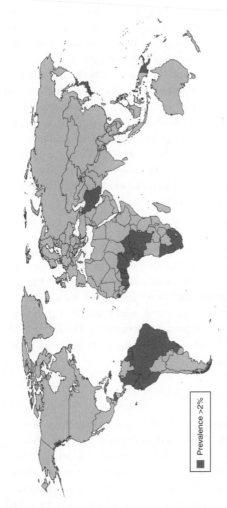

15. World map showing the prevalence of HTLV-1 infection

■ Prevalence >2%

difficult to treat, and rapidly fatal. ATL is an adult disease, but almost all patients suffering from it acquired the virus from their mothers in infancy, indicating that the disease requires a long incubation period. This suggests that HTLV-1 infection is only one of a series of cellular events that lead to ATL. Studies have identified HTLV-1's 'tax' gene as the major transforming gene. This codes for the 'tax' protein that has a multitude of functions including driving cell proliferation, decreasing cell death, and increasing virus replication. One particularly important function is the production of a self-stimulatory growth loop that causes the cell to produce the T cell growth factor, interleukin-2. At the same time, it up-regulates the expression of the T cell growth factor's receptor on the cell surface. All these functions enhance the survival of the virus by increasing the number of infected cells in the body and also increase the chance of random mutations occurring in infected cells.

There are no very effective treatments for ATL, and no vaccine against HTLV-1 that would prevent infection. However, in most countries, blood for transfusion is routinely screened for HTLV-1, so blocking this route of spread. In addition, most mother to child transmission can be prevented by antenatal testing and advising HTLV-positive mothers not to breast feed. This test is in place in Japan, but its effect on incidence of ATL will not be evident for several decades.

The herpesviruses

As we have seen in Chapter 6, herpesviruses form a very widespread and highly successful family, having evolved mechanisms to evade immune responses and persist in their hosts for life. By far the majority of these persistent infections are 'silent', or asymptomatic, but occasionally problems may arise. For a significant number of herpesviruses that infect humans and other vertebrates these include tumour development.

Of the eight known human herpesviruses, two are oncogenic – Epstein–Barr virus (EBV) and Kaposi sarcoma-associated herpesvirus (KSHV). Both viruses spread by close contact, mainly by salivary contact during childhood. Among adults, KSHV spreads by the sexual route, especially between male homosexual partners, and there is some evidence that EBV can also be spread sexually. These viruses both establish latency in blood B cells. EBV also replicates in epithelial cells lining mucosal surfaces and KSHV in endothelial cells lining blood vessels.

Relative to other viruses, herpesviruses are large, coding for between 70 and 100 genes, and both EBV and KSHV carry their own set of latent genes that induce cell proliferation. It is thought that expression of these genes helps the virus establish a persistent infection in the body. Some of the latent genes are viral oncogenes, but unlike retroviruses that have transduced their oncogenes from their host genome, these are unique to the virus. These oncogenes interfere with cellular control mechanisms, driving cell proliferation, and enhance the virus's long-term survival.

Both EBV and KSHV cause tumours that are geographically restricted, suggesting the involvement of local co-factors. People whose immune systems are suppressed are also at risk of tumours caused by these viruses because they are incapable of controlling the latent virus infection.

EBV was discovered in 1964 after the London-based virologist Anthony Epstein spent two years searching for a virus in biopsy material from Burkitt lymphoma (BL). BL, the commonest childhood tumour in central Africa, was first described by a British surgeon, Denis Burkitt, in 1958, while working in Uganda. The tumour, which is composed of B cells, mainly targets children between the ages of 7 and 14 and is more common in boys. The clinical presentation is striking, with fast-growing swellings, most often around the jaw, and it is rapidly fatal if untreated. Burkitt mapped the geography of the tumour to low-lying areas in equatorial

Africa where the rainfall exceeded 55 cm per year and the
temperature did not fall below 16°C (Figure 16). Because of this tight
geographic restriction, Epstein proposed an infectious cause for
the tumour and began his search. He and his graduate student,
Yvonne Barr, eventually isolated the new herpesvirus that now bears
their names from cultured BL cells. But it soon became apparent
that this was a ubiquitous virus, making it difficult to prove that it
caused a tumour restricted to children in central Africa.

We now know that BL is also common in the coastal regions
of Papua New Guinea and that around 97% of all tropical

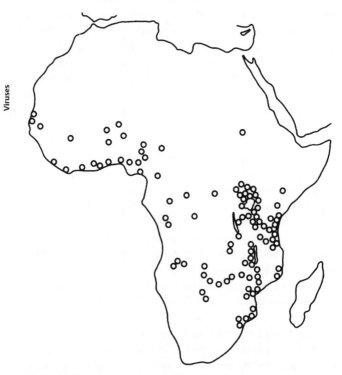

16. Burkitt's map of the distribution of Burkitt's lymphoma in Africa

BL tumours contain EBV. BL also occurs at low incidence in temperate regions, where only around 25% of tumours are EBV-associated. Surprisingly, the viral oncogenes are not expressed in BL cells, so the role of EBV in cell transformation is unclear. In contrast, a cellular genetic abnormality is present in all BL tumour cells whether EBV-associated or not. This involves a chromosome translocation that moves a cellular oncogene called c-myc from its normal place on chromosome 8 to another location. In doing so, this deregulates the oncogene, and it causes uncontrolled cell proliferation, clearly an important step in tumour development.

The local climatic conditions for BL in Africa as defined by Burkitt also apply in New Guinea and mirror those of year-round malaria infection. For malaria, these conditions are determined by the breeding requirements of its vector, the mosquito. EBV is not spread by mosquitoes, but it seems that malaria is an added risk factor for the development of BL, perhaps because the associated chronic inflammation enhances the survival and proliferation of EBV-infected B cells. However, we still don't know exactly how malaria infection, c-myc deregulation, and EBV infection act together to promote tumour development.

Interestingly, there is an increased incidence of BL in AIDS patients around the globe, but only about one-quarter of these tumours contain EBV. This suggests that HIV infection with its associated immunosuppression and chronic inflammation can replace the need for EBV and malaria in tumour development.

The situation is much clearer for EBV-associated tumours that occur in people whose immunity is suppressed either because of a congenital immune defect or immunosuppressive drugs like those taken by transplant recipients to prevent the rejection of their grafted organ. Suppression of T cell immunity in particular allows EBV-infected cells expressing viral oncogenes to survive and proliferate, sometimes causing a tumour. This seems a very direct form of tumour production, but the fact that only a minority of immunosuppressed people develop tumours suggests that additional factors, presumably cellular mutations, are required for tumour growth.

EBV is also found in around 50% of cases of Hodgkin's lymphoma, particularly those in children in developing countries, in people with HIV, and in elderly Caucasians, as well as epithelial tumours of the nasal mucosa called nasopharyngeal carcinoma which are very common in southern China, and in around 10–20% of stomach cancers.

Kaposi sarcoma-associated virus was discovered in 1994 by husband and wife team Yuang Chan and Patrick Moore in Pittsburgh, USA, after a search prompted by the epidemic of Kaposi sarcoma (KS) in people infected with HIV. KS occurs in three forms, the first being the 'classic' form described by Austro-Hungarian dermatologist Moritz Kaposi (1837–1902) in 1872. This characteristically presents as multiple reddish-brown patches on the skin of elderly men of Mediterranean, Eastern European, or Jewish origin. It is slow-growing and only rarely invades internal organs. The second is the 'endemic' form of KS that is found in East Africa and is similar to the classic form but invasion of internal organs is more common. The third KS type is 'AIDS-associated' and was initially very common in gay men in the West, but while its incidence there has declined following the introduction of retroviral therapy for HIV, it has increased in sub-Saharan Africa, where it is now the commonest HIV-associated tumour.

KS lesions are composed of KSHV-infected endothelial cells known as spindle cells. In addition, the virus produces factors that stimulate excessive new blood vessel formation, giving the tumour its characteristic red colouration. The viral genome contains oncogenes and also growth factor and growth factor receptor genes, all of which stimulate tumour cell proliferation. KSHV also causes the rare B cell tumours multicentric Castleman's disease and primary effusion lymphoma. All these tumour types occur more commonly with immunosuppression.

Hepatitis viruses

Primary liver cancer is a major global health problem, being one of the ten most common cancers worldwide, with over 250,000 cases diagnosed every year and only 5% of sufferers surviving 5 years. The tumour is more common in men than women and is most prevalent in sub-Saharan Africa and South-East Asia where the incidence reaches over 30 per 100,000 population per year, compared to fewer than 5 per 100,000 in the USA and Europe. Up to 80% of these tumours are caused by a hepatitis virus, the remainder being related to liver damage from toxic agents such as alcohol.

As we have seen in the previous chapter, there are five human hepatitis viruses (A, B, C, D, and E), of which hepatitis B and C viruses cause liver cancer. These two viruses are unrelated to each other, HBV being a small DNA hepadnavirus, whereas HCV is a flavivirus with an RNA genome. However, both primarily attack the liver, causing either overt hepatitis or a silent infection on first encounter. In some people, they persist, often causing continued liver damage, cirrhosis, and, in the unfortunate few, liver cancer.

The association between HBV and liver cancer is supported by the geographical co-incidence between the highest levels of virus infection and tumour occurrence; these occur in South America, sub-Saharan Africa, and South-East Asia (Figure 14). In addition, a large study carried out on 22,000 men in Taiwan in the 1990s showed that those persistently infected with HBV were over 200 times more likely than non-carriers to develop liver cancer, and that over half the deaths in this group were due to liver cancer or cirrhosis.

However, the mechanism of tumour development by HBV is not entirely clear. Since the tumour develops many years after the initial infection, several rare events must be required for tumour outgrowth. The virus does not code for any proteins that transform liver cells in tissue culture or induce tumours in animals, but it carries a gene called X that can activate cellular genes and may therefore influence the cell's growth control mechanisms. Also, the majority of tumours contain one or more copies of the HBV genome integrated into cellular DNA. This integration is randomly sited and probably occurs as an accident during division of an HBV-infected cell since, unlike retroviruses, integration is not part of HBV's natural life cycle. This event may occur on several occasions over a lifelong infection, but can only promote tumour development if the site of integration allows the X gene to influence cellular genes, tipping the balance in favour of cell growth. In addition, the chronic inflammation caused by persistent infection of liver cells, with recurring cycles of cell infection, immune destruction, and liver cell regeneration which sometimes lead to cirrhosis, may provide growth factors that aid tumour growth. Finally, certain toxins that may contaminate poorly preserved food can cause liver cancers in animals. Aflotoxin B1 produced by fungi is one such example that may therefore act as another unrelated co-factor for the disease in humans.

A vaccine against HBV is available, and its use has already caused a decline in HBV-related liver cancer in Taiwan, where a vaccination programme was implemented in the 1980s (see Chapter 8).

Similar to HBV, persistent HCV infection is associated with the risk of primary liver cancer, and in countries where the rates of liver cancer have recently fallen thanks to an HBV vaccination programme targeted at high-risk groups, HCV is now the commonest cause of this fatal disease.

The mechanism of HCV tumour development is far from clear, and the fact that the virus could not be grown in culture until recently severely hampered research programmes. Importantly, though, extensive searching of tumour tissue has failed to find any trace of the virus, and no transforming viral genes have been identified. These facts suggest that the role of the virus in tumour development is entirely indirect. Perhaps the chronic inflammatory processes stimulated by the virus over decades are enough on rare occasions to trigger malignant change.

Papilloma viruses

Nearly everyone has suffered from unsightly warts on the hands or painful verrucae on the soles of the feet at some time in their lives. These are caused by human papilloma viruses (HPVs), a very large family of viruses with over 100 different types. Infection with HPVs is very common and although most, like those causing warts and verrucae, are harmless, a few types can cause cancer, most commonly cancer of the uterine cervix in women.

Skin warts caused by a papilloma virus were first described in the 1930s by Richard Shope, who worked alongside Payton Rous at the Rockefeller Institute in New York. He decided to follow up on a story told to him by game hunters suggesting that rabbits in Iowa had horns. The horns turned out to be warty skin tumours from which Shope was able to extract a filterable agent that caused the same warty lesions when painted onto the skin of healthy rabbits. These sometimes developed into invasive tumours. However, in those days, he could only speculate as to the type of virus that caused these lesions.

We now know that HPVs target squamous epithelial cells, that is, the thick layer of cells that make up the skin on the outside of our bodies, and line certain internal areas such as the genital tract, the mouth, the throat, and upper larynx. The basal layer of the epithelium contains self-renewing stem cells capable of a lifetime of cell division. This production line is normally finely balanced by cell loss from the regular shedding of dead cells from the skin surface. Entering through a small cut or abrasion, HPVs set up a persistent infection in these epithelial stem cells. The HPV genome replicates each time the cell divides, with one copy being retained in the stem cell offspring so ensuring its long-term survival in the host. The second daughter cell progresses up the epithelium, and its maturation is the signal for HPV to begin virus production, so that when the cell dies and is shed from the surface, it contains thousands of virus particles ready to infect new hosts, spread by close contact such as sexual intercourse.

The link between HPV and cervical cancer was suggested in the 1970s by Harald zur Hausen, a German virologist from Nuremberg who then went on to prove the association and win a Nobel Prize for his discovery in 2008. We now know that HPV DNA, particularly from types 16 and 18, is present in the cells of almost all cervical cancers, as well as the less common cancers of the skin, mouth, throat, and larynx.

The HPV DNA genome is small, with just eight or nine major genes. In natural infection, the role of genes called E6 and E7 is to drive the cell to divide so that the virus has access to the cellular machinery it needs to propagate its own genome. Thus HPV-infected cells often grow faster than uninfected cells, resulting in the typical small cauliflower-like shape of a wart. However, this on its own does not lead to cancer; for a malignant change to occur other factors are required, particularly integration of the viral genome into that of the host cell. This, like HBV integration, is a rare and random occurrence that presumably results from a mistake during cell division. It deregulates viral gene expression, leading to overexpression of E6 and E7 and an increased rate of cell division.

These laboratory findings are backed up by the clinical observation of HPV types 16 and 18 in the cervix of some women not suffering from cancer. Indeed, tests on 18- to 25-year-old healthy American women show that up to 46% carry HPV, of which types 16 and 18 account for around one-third. Furthermore, regular screening for cervical cancer set up in the 1960s identified precancerous lesions where the abnormal, virus-infected cells remain within the epithelium layer. This is called cervical intra-epithelial neoplasia (CIN) and is graded on a severity scale of I to III. HPV DNA is present in all grades, and although regression back to normal may occur at any stage, a large percentage of untreated stages II and III progress to invasive cancer.

Factors that increase the chances of HPV infection and genital cancer include young age at first sexual intercourse, high numbers of sexual partners, use of oral contraceptives, and other sexually transmitted infections. Once infected, the risk of cancer development is higher in those who smoke, the immunosuppressed, and women with an affected relative, the latter indicating a genetic predisposition to the disease.

Unfortunately, although cervical screening can pick out those infected with high-risk HPV types and follow the progression of CIN, at the present time it cannot definitively predict who will develop overt cancer. In addition, the procedure is too expensive to implement in developing countries, where the risk of cervical cancer may be high.

The incidence of cancer of the cervix varies from one country to another, with the highest incidences in South Africa and Central America, where it is the commonest cancer diagnosed in women (Figure 17). Worldwide, there are nearly half a million new cases and over quarter of a million deaths annually from cervical cancer. Although the incidence and death rates have fallen in the Western world since the introduction of screening, this is not the case in developing countries, which now account for 85% of the total. A vaccine against HPV 16 and 18 is now being offered to teenage girls in the USA, UK, and Continental Europe (see Chapter 8) in the belief that preventing infection with the two most oncogenic

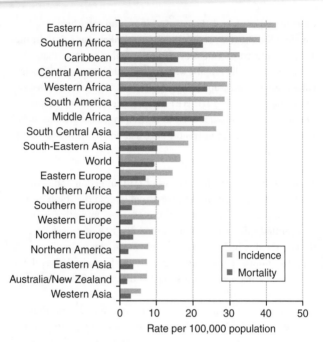

17. **Age-standardized incidence and mortality rates for cervical cancer by world region, 2002 estimates**

HPVs will have a dramatic effect on the incidence of cancer of the cervix in years to come. As the vaccine is cheaper and easier to administer than cervical screening, it is hoped that it will soon reach the countries with the greatest need.

Hit and run?

Presently, 1.8 million virus-associated cancers are diagnosed worldwide annually. This accounts for 18% of all cancers, but since these human tumour viruses were only identified fairly recently, it is probable that there are several more out there waiting to be discovered. If this is the case, then it is important to find them because a viral cause opens up the possibility of a vaccine to prevent the tumour.

KSHV is the most recently discovered human tumour virus, and this was detected using molecular probes rather than traditional virus isolation methods. Yuang and Moore compared DNA from a KS lesion with DNA from normal skin of the same individual in a subtraction experiment. They eliminated all the identical DNA sequences in the two samples, leaving only DNA sequences unique to KS, and these turned out to be DNA sequences from an undiscovered herpesvirus – KSHV. This clever technological trick is being applied to other tumours suspected of a viral cause, but for some the result might not be very encouraging. A mechanism known as 'hit and run' has been suggested whereby the culprit virus acts early in tumour development, permanently damaging the cell, and then departs to leave no trace. If this is the mechanism used, then it will certainly be difficult to prove an association between viruses and cancer.

Chapter 8
Turning the tables

It is curiously paradoxical that the prevention of several virus infections was achieved long before anyone knew of the existence of viruses or of the immune responses required to prevent infection. Whereas viruses were first recognized in the 1930s, over 100 years before this, Edward Jenner (1749–1823) succeeded in vaccinating against smallpox, the biggest killer virus of all time.

Smallpox prevention and eradication

The first recorded way of preventing smallpox was inoculation, used in China and India for hundreds of years before it reached Western Europe in the 1700s. The technique, also called variolation or engraftment, involved scratching the skin with a needle dipped in scrapings or pus from a smallpox lesion. Unlike virus acquired by inhalation, this generally produced a localized skin infection but no systemic infection and was followed by long-term immunity.

Inoculation was introduced to Britain in the 1720s by Lady Mary Wortley Montagu (1689–1762), who saw it performed while living in Constantinople (now Istanbul) with her husband, Edward Wortley Montagu, the British ambassador to the Ottoman Empire from 1716 to 1717. Lady Mary had suffered from smallpox herself and her brother had died of the disease, so she was willing to try anything that might protect her children. She persuaded the family physician, Dr Charles Maitland, to learn the technique from local practitioners in Constantinople and then inoculate her 5-year-old son Edward. This he did, and a week later the child developed fever with a few pocks but soon recovered and was then immune.

When the family returned to London in 1718, Lady Mary was keen to publicize inoculation as a way of preventing smallpox, and when an epidemic broke out in 1721, she asked Maitland to inoculate her daughter Mary, aged 4, with two eminent physicians as witnesses. This was successfully accomplished, and the word spread. After further inoculations were carried out on six criminals from Newgate Prison and a group of orphans from London's Parish of St James without ill effect, King George I gave consent for his two granddaughters to be inoculated, so popularizing the technique. However, inoculation was bitterly opposed by many of the clergy, who felt that it went against the will of God, and by some doctors who foresaw a loss of income. Others genuinely feared that it might cause smallpox, sparking an epidemic among the non-immune. Indeed, inoculation did sometimes cause full-blown smallpox and had a mortality rate of 1–2%, but this compares with a 10–20% death rate from smallpox among the un-inoculated. The technique was used widely in Europe and the USA until the safer method of vaccination was introduced at the beginning of the 19th century.

Edward Jenner was a country doctor from Berkeley, Gloucestershire, UK, where it was rumoured that milkmaids' unblemished skin was due to contracting cowpox, a natural infection of cows' udders, and thereafter being immune from smallpox. These rumours possibly stemmed from Benjamin Jesty (1736–1816), a farmer from Dorset, who was probably the first to test this theory, in 1774, when he inoculated his wife and children with cowpox, but he did not pursue the experiment any further. It is not clear whether Jenner knew of Jesty's work before he decided to test the theory for himself, but he later acknowledged Jesty's contribution.

Jenner went for the most direct proof possible. In his now world-famous experiments, which by today's standards would not proceed on ethical grounds, he obtained cowpox from the arm of an infected milkmaid, Sarah Nelmes, and used it to inoculate a child, James Phipps, who had not had smallpox. A few weeks later, he inoculated Phipps with live smallpox to see if he was protected. Fortunately, Phipps remained healthy, and when several other children tested with cowpox were also protected from smallpox, Jenner knew he had made a groundbreaking discovery that had the potential to save many thousands of lives.

However, when Jenner published his findings in a pamphlet in 1798, others were not so sure. Some did not believe that vaccination would work. They advised Jenner, who had been elected a Fellow of the Royal Society for his discovery that cuckoos lay their eggs in other birds' nests, to stick to his original ornithological research. He also encountered opposition from the church similar to that experienced by Lady Mary, further strengthened by a public outcry against the use of animals (cows) to prevent a disease in humans (Figure 18). But despite this opposition, the use of smallpox vaccination, which was safer than inoculation, spread rapidly, and by 1801 more than 100,000 people in the UK had been vaccinated. Over the following 50 years, deaths from smallpox in London fell from over 90 to 15 per 1,000.

At first, cowpox virus for vaccination was obtained from naturally infected cows or milkmaids, but arm-to-arm passage from inoculated to non-immune people was soon developed, and later the virus was grown on, and harvested from, the flanks of cows, a method more suited to large-scale production. The practice of vaccination remains almost unchanged to the present day and was essential for worldwide smallpox eradication.

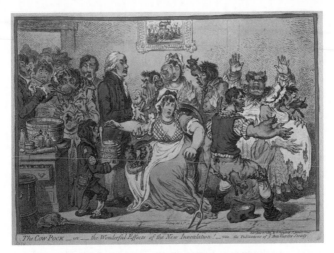

18. 'The Cow-Pock-or-The Wonderful Effects of the New Inoculation', by James Gillray, 1802

By 1966, when the WHO announced the Smallpox Eradication Campaign, the virus had already been eliminated from Europe and the USA, but was still endemic in 31 countries, giving an estimated 10 million cases and 2 million deaths annually. The campaign was predicted to be costly, but as the disease was so deadly, even countries that had eliminated the virus lived in fear of imported cases causing an epidemic and so were willing to provide funds for global eradication.

The success of this bold, highly complex, and expensive endeavour critically depended on several specific features of the smallpox virus, the disease itself, and the vaccine. Firstly, the virus has no animal reservoir; it only infects humans, causing an acute illness with no virus persistence in survivors. So as the virus has nowhere to hide, interruption of its chain of infection should eventually lead to its elimination. Secondly, that this disease was non-infectious until the symptoms appeared, when they were severe enough to keep the patient relatively isolated in bed. The disease itself was easy to diagnose from the clinical features, particularly the characteristic rash. So since no silent infections occurred, virtually all cases could be identified and isolated. Furthermore, the incubation period of around two weeks provided a window of opportunity for chasing the contacts of a case and isolating them until they were deemed non-infectious. Thirdly, that the vaccine, which was absolutely key to the success of the campaign, was safe and highly effective. And as smallpox virus is a stable DNA virus with only the one major type, there was little likelihood of it mutating into a vaccine-resistant strain.

A vaccine preparation that remained active in tropical climates was produced and distributed by armies of workers in the world's four remaining endemic zones: Brazil, Indonesia, sub-Saharan Africa, and the Indian subcontinent. The aim was to increase vaccination coverage to over 80%, the critical level for preventing virus spread. This worked so well that within 10 years smallpox transmission was finally interrupted, Ethiopia being the last endemic country. Worldwide, eradication of smallpox was declared in 1980.

Amazingly, the last two cases of smallpox worldwide occurred in the UK in 1978. These were related to ongoing smallpox virus research in the Department of Microbiology at the University of Birmingham Medical School where one victim, a photographer in the Anatomy Department, died and another who caught the disease from her recovered. The Anatomy Department was situated on the floor above the microbiology laboratories, and the enquiry that followed the disaster found that the conditions used to contain the virus in the laboratory were 'far from satisfactory'. The report suggested that the virus had travelled via air ducts from the virus preparation area to a phone box in the Anatomy Department on the floor above that was often used by the photographer. The whole incident had a final upsetting outcome when the Head of the Microbiology Department committed suicide following the enquiry's highly critical report of the Department's safety procedures.

Jenner's vaccine works by generating an immune response to a harmless virus (cowpox) that is so closely related to the lethal virus (smallpox) that the immune system cannot distinguish between the two. This same trick was later used to prevent Marek's disease, a devastating infection of poultry caused by a tumour-associated herpesvirus called Marek's disease virus. It mainly affects chickens and rapidly kills up to 80% of a domestic flock, causing severe financial loss. The disease, first described by Hungarian pathologist Jozef Marek (1868–1952) in 1907, begins with paralysis of one or more limbs followed by difficulty in breathing leading to death. These symptoms are caused by T cells infiltrating the nerves and producing tumours in vital organs. Once the virus was isolated in 1967, it was soon discovered that a very similar virus, herpesvirus of turkeys, could protect chickens from Marek's disease virus without ill effect.

Rabies vaccination

Several years after Jenner's experiments, Louis Pasteur, working in Paris, made a vaccine against rabies virus from dried spinal cords of rabies-infected animals. This virus is present in saliva from rabid animals and generally circulates among wild animals such as dogs, foxes, and bats. Although some species can survive an attack of rabies, untreated human infections, usually acquired through the bite of a rabid dog, are 100% fatal. Death results from the virus invading the brain, but not before it has induced the most distressing symptoms. These include the classic hydrophobia (fear of water) combined with periods of extreme excitement and hyper-activity interspersed by lucid intervals when the patient is all too aware of their desperate plight. Patients experience terrifying spasms of their respiratory muscles when trying to drink, but thirst drives them to repeated attempts to drink, with violent effects that may lead to generalized convulsions and cardiac or respiratory arrest. Otherwise, patients survive in this state for about a week before sinking into a coma and dying. It is no wonder that Pasteur chose rabies as the first infectious disease he attempted to prevent with a vaccine.

In 1885, while his vaccine was still being tested in the laboratory, Pasteur was persuaded to try it out on a child, Joseph Meister, who had been badly bitten by a rabid dog and whose outlook was grim. The vaccine saved the child's life, and many others thereafter, until it was replaced by a safer preparation made by growing the virus in cultured cells.

Unlike vaccines designed to prevent acute infections such as measles and polio, rabies vaccine can protect from the disease even if it is given after the bite that transmits the virus. This is known as 'post-exposure' vaccination. This is because the virus must follow nerve pathways from the site of infection to the brain before causing symptoms. The journey may take months or even years, the duration depending on the distance between the site of infection and the brain. So as long as the vaccine is given soon after the bite, it should prevent the virus reaching the brain. Although relatively rare, rabies is endemic in most of the world, with up to 70,000 deaths annually from the disease globally, the highest annual death rate recorded in one country being 20,000 in India. Vaccination is recommended if travelling in countries with a high incidence, but in practice post-exposure vaccination is in high demand, with over 13 million doses given annually.

There is no doubt that although vaccines are expensive to prepare and test, they are the safest, easiest, and most cost-effective way of controlling infectious diseases worldwide. For this reason, vaccines against almost every pathogenic virus from the common cold virus to the highly lethal Ebola virus are currently in preparation. But vaccine development is a long-drawn-out process, and although several are in clinical trials, relatively few have been licensed for clinical use. These include a triple vaccine for the once common childhood illnesses, measles, mumps, and rubella, given by two injections, one at 13 months and one at 3 to 5 years of age.

Traditionally, there are two types of viral vaccines, one using live attenuated (weakened) virus and the other inactivated virus. The pros and cons of using these different vaccines are illustrated by the story of polio eradication, which has now entered its end game.

During the early 1900s, polio was a much-feared disease (see Chapter 5). Epidemics reached a peak in the USA in the 1950s, just before the inactivated vaccine produced by American virologist Jonas Salk (1914–95) came into use. It had an immediate effect, reducing the number of polio cases in the USA from 20,000 to around 2,000 per year. However, it had to be given by injection, and at first it was of fairly low potency.

For these reasons, another American virologist, Albert Sabin (1906–93), manufactured a live attenuated polio vaccine that became available in the early 1960s. He grew the virus in the laboratory until a weakened strain emerged that induced immunity without causing disease. This vaccine was cheaper and easier to produce than the inactivated product and could be taken orally, a great advantage, particularly for use in the developing world. Furthermore, oral administration uses the natural route of wild polio virus infection, and so the vaccine strain replicates in the gut and is excreted in faeces. It can then spread in the community, effectively vaccinating those who have not officially received a dose of vaccine. However, because the virus grows in the body, there is a chance that it will mutate into a pathogenic strain. Although rare, this does occur, with live attenuated polio vaccine causing paralytic polio in about one in a million vaccinees.

The WHO Polio World Eradication Campaign begun in 1988 aimed to achieve over 80% coverage with oral vaccine. This was highly successful in eradicating wild virus, and the global incidence had declined by 99% by 2005, with just a few pockets of infection remaining in Afghanistan, India, Pakistan, and Nigeria. Paradoxically, as the incidence of wild polio infection declined, the relative risk of vaccine-related polio caused by mutant vaccine virus rose, so that now most cases of paralytic polio are caused by the vaccine strain. Also, with the vaccine strain of polio virus circulating in the community, it is not possible to completely eradicate the virus. For these reasons, several Western countries have reverted to using the inactivated vaccine, and this will probably have to happen worldwide before complete eradication can be achieved.

Other human viruses on the list for worldwide eradication include measles, rubella, mumps, rabies, and HBV.

To vaccinate or not to vaccinate?

The ethical debate surrounding the use of smallpox vaccination in Jenner's time has moved on but certainly not disappeared. There are still religious sects who refuse vaccination, but other major issues have now come to the fore.

One of these is the 'hygiene hypothesis' invoked to explain the recent rise in autoimmune and allergic diseases in Western countries. Both these types of disease are caused by an imbalance in the immune response. The hygiene theory attributes this to a lack of childhood infections resulting from vaccinations as well as rising standards of hygiene and antibiotic use in the modern world. All these factors decrease antigenic stimulation during childhood and could predispose a child's immune system to these abnormal responses. Research in this field continues, but at the time of writing, there is no concrete evidence to support the hypothesis.

However safe vaccines are, they will never be completely without potential side effects. As they continue to succeed in preventing infectious diseases, so death rates will fall, and eventually the adverse effects of a vaccine may exceed those of the disease it was designed to prevent. Although the risks of smallpox vaccine are exceedingly small, at one or two deaths per million vaccinations, this was bound to happen at some point during the smallpox eradication programme as the virus was banished from whole continents. Even so, it was still essential that vaccination continued until complete eradication was ensured. At the present time, while global eradication of measles is ongoing, and infection is now a rare event in the developed world, some may think that with a one in a million risk of vaccine-associated encephalitis, it is safer not to vaccinate. However, if enough people argue this way and the level of vaccination falls below the critical level of 80%, then measles epidemics will reappear, leading inevitably to deaths.

This is exactly what happened in the UK after a report appeared in the medical journal *The Lancet* in 1998 suggesting a link between measles vaccination and childhood autism. The publicity this received caused an immediate downturn in measles vaccinations and, despite the link being refuted and eventually disproved, the dip lasted long enough for the virus to re-establish itself in the community and cause measles epidemics and deaths. It took 12 years for the report's senior author, Andrew Wakefield, to be found guilty of dishonesty and flouting ethics protocols by the General Medical Council and to be struck off the UK Medical Register. Only then did *The Lancet* officially retract the report on the basis of false claims of ethical approval.

For all these reasons, there is a constant search for safer vaccines. The molecular revolution beginning in the 1960s heralded a new generation of recombinant subunit viral vaccines. With the molecular makeup of viruses finally unravelled, the key viral proteins (subunits) required to stimulate protective immunity could be identified and manufactured in the laboratory as a vaccine. The first of these new recombinant vaccines to come on line was against HBV. HBV surface antigen was identified as the key protein, and this was cloned and produced in vast quantities in yeast cells in the laboratory. After animal experiments showed the vaccine to be safe and effective, it replaced earlier products made by purifying HBV surface antigen from the blood of persistently infected individuals, a practice that carried the risk of also transferring blood-borne infections such as HIV and HCV. A similar laboratory-based product is the recently licensed vaccine against the cancer-causing HPV types 16 and 18 based on the major viral coat protein. These HPV protein molecules are assembled into hollow, non-infectious 'virus-like particles' that have been shown, using animal models, to be safe and to prevent HPV-induced cancer development. The vaccine is now recommended for teenage girls to prevent cancer of the cervix.

Other modern inventions using recombinant vaccines are so-called naked DNA vaccines, for which the DNA that codes for the key viral protein is either injected directly or inserted into the genome of a harmless virus for delivery. When this virus, called a vector, infects human or animal cells, it expresses the key 'foreign' gene along with its own genes and generates a host immune response. No vaccines made in this way have yet been granted a licence for human use, but clinical trials have been carried out on a recombinant HIV vaccine using an adenovirus as a vector.

Despite these varied approaches to vaccine production, there are still many pathogenic viruses with no available vaccines, including the childhood killer respiratory syncytial virus. There are a variety of reasons for this, which are illustrated by the many failed attempts to prepare a vaccine against HIV.

HIV vaccines: fact or fiction?

It is now over 20 years since HIV was first identified as the cause of AIDS, but despite massive financial investment and scientific effort, there is no effective vaccine on the horizon. After HIV vaccine preparations that primarily stimulated antibody responses failed to prevent infection, T cell vaccines were tried, but these too have failed – one even seemed to increase infection rates in the vaccinated group compared to the controls.

There are several reasons for these failures. Firstly, HIV mutates rapidly, and after around 100 years of human infection there are many different types and strains that may not all be prevented by a single vaccine preparation. Secondly, HIV persists in everyone it infects, indicating that the natural immune response against it cannot clear the virus. This makes it tough to design a vaccine that will do what nature cannot achieve. Thirdly, HIV is usually transmitted via the lining of the genital tract, so antibodies and immune T cells in the blood must reach this site to prevent HIV infecting CD4 cells and establishing latent infection. Finally, HIV may be transmitted either as free virus or inside cells such that the immune response required to prevent it establishing infection in each case may be different. For all these reasons, the ideal vaccine that prevents HIV infection entirely is at present a remote possibility. Even a vaccine that controls the infection and prolongs the disease-free period would be helpful. A slight glimmer of hope came in 2009 when the results of the largest and most expensive HIV vaccine trial to date were announced. The trial, involving 16,000 volunteers in Thailand, took six years to complete and was generally expected to fail. However, the results showed a modest level of protection produced by two recombinant vaccines given in a 'prime-boost' scenario. The first shot was designed to stimulate a T cell response to HIV and the second to boost this response.

Even if this is the beginning of a breakthrough for HIV vaccines, a licensed product is still a long way off. In the meantime, other ways of tackling the deadly infection must be used to maximum effect.

The multifaceted approach to controlling HIV still focuses on interrupting spread of the virus but goes beyond the traditional means of education, free access to condoms, and needle-exchange programmes and prompt treatment of other sexually transmitted infections. For instance, circumcision has been shown to reduce the risk of infection in men by 40–80% and is therefore to be encouraged in certain high-risk groups.

Antiviral drugs are key in curtailing viral spread and are being rolled out worldwide, with present coverage of around 50% of those in need. A priority area is to deliver antiretroviral drugs to all HIV-positive pregnant women to prevent virus transfer to the child, and this is expected to be implemented by 2015.

Taking a leaf out of the malaria prevention book, where pre-exposure prophylaxis is the norm, one option is to protect high-risk, uninfected partners of HIV-infected people with antiretroviral drugs. In addition, the post-exposure prophylaxis used successfully in healthcare workers after accidental occupational HIV exposure is an option following high-risk sexual encounters, mirroring the thinking behind the night-after contraceptive pill.

Many studies show that HIV transmission occurs most readily when the viral load in the blood is high, and since antiviral therapy can reduce this load to undetectable levels, these drugs can be used to prevent spread. Most transmission occurs in the few months following primary infection when the viral load is extremely high but when most people are unaware of their infection. More effective screening programmes of at-risk groups, including opt-out testing, would pick up these early infections and allow early treatment.

Antiviral agents

For almost 40 years after the discovery of penicillin in 1945, bacterial infections could be cured with the appropriate antibiotic, while most virus infections were untreatable. This contrast relates to the biological differences between bacteria and viruses and in the way they cause disease. Pathogenic bacteria are mostly free-living, single-celled organisms that can invade and multiply in the body, so causing disease. Bacteria have tough outer cell walls that are essential for their survival, and penicillin and its derivatives target these unique structures while leaving host cells unharmed. However, viruses are not cells, and because they use the replication machinery of the cells they infect, it has proved difficult to find drugs that prevent virus replication without damaging the host. Despite this, there are now almost 40 antiviral drugs approved for clinical use. Unfortunately, most are only active against a single virus or virus group.

The first antiviral drug to be licensed was aciclovir, made in the 1970s and active against herpesvirus infections such as cold sores and shingles. The drug masquerades as a nucleoside, the building block of DNA. In order to be incorporated into herpesvirus DNA, phosphate groups must be added to each nucleoside by a herpesvirus enzyme called thymidine kinase. This essential step restricts the drug's activity to virus-infected cells. Phosphorylated aciclovir then joins the growing viral DNA chain and blocks its extension, so terminating viral DNA replication. By targeting a virus-specific function, in this case replication of its DNA, aciclovir spares uninfected host cells and therefore does no collateral damage.

The recognition of HIV as the cause of AIDS in the early 1980s gave a much needed impetus to antiviral drug discovery. Now around half of the licensed antiretroviral compounds are specifically designed for HIV treatment and have transformed a uniformly fatal infection into a chronic disease. Many antiretroviral compounds act in a similar way to aciclovir by inhibiting viral enzymes essential for viral replication, in this case targeting HIV's reverse transcriptase, protease, or integrase enzymes. Other drugs inhibit HIV's entry into cells. But since HIV mutates frequently, it rapidly generates resistance to a single drug. In 1996, it became apparent that a cocktail of at least three drugs of different classes (called highly active antiretroviral therapy, HAART) was superior to single drug therapy. Whilst lifelong control of HIV can only be achieved by strict adherence to this regimen, with the drug combination changed at the first sign of resistance (usually a rising viral load) or if side effects become intolerable, most HIV-infected people taking HAART have a normal life expectancy.

Flu is another infection that can be treated with a variety of antiviral drugs. These are based on two modes of action: one inhibits the virus's neuraminidase enzyme and the other blocks virus entry into host cells. During the short course of treatment required to cure flu, drug resistance is not generally a problem, but in an epidemic or pandemic situation it may be. As we saw in the 2009 H1N1 swine flu pandemic, the drug Tamiflu (Oseltamivir, which is a neuraminidase inhibitor) was stockpiled by many governments in developed countries. This worked fine at the beginning of the pandemic, but then resistant strains began to circulate. The hope was that the drug would fill the gap while a vaccine was prepared. This approach worked reasonably well, particularly for severe cases. However, since the pandemic flu strain turned out to be generally mild, the strategy was not really put to the test.

Clearance of persistent hepatitis viruses

On a worldwide scale, persistent HBV and HCV are an enormous problem, accounting for around 250,000 deaths annually. And yet some people clear these viruses after primary infection, so treatment aims to induce clearance in those who suffer persistent active infection. At present, this is not always possible, but the combination of antiviral drugs and immune stimulants can often suppress virus replication and restrict liver damage.

The cytokine interferon-α has both immune-stimulating and antiviral effects and is used for treatment of both viruses. However, there is a serious downside. The treatment involves a long course of injections with some unpleasant side effects, mostly flu-like symptoms with lethargy. It also sometimes causes depression, and around 15% of patients are unable to complete the course.

Used as a single therapy, interferon-α gives a sustained response in up to 40% of people with persistent HBV infection, and similar results are obtained with single antiviral drugs. The latter are presently the treatment of choice, but clinical trials are in progress to assess the role of combining interferon-α with antiviral drugs for HBV management. Persistent HCV also responds to interferon-α, and a response rate of up to 80% is obtained when this is combined with antiviral drugs. The outcome depends on infecting HCV subtype, the extent of the disease, and the age and sex of the patient. The best results are achieved in individuals with subtypes 2, 3, or 4 and a low viral load.

Virus diagnosis

Historically, diagnosis and treatment of virus infections have lagged far behind those of bacterial diseases and are only now catching up. Originally, viruses were identified as infectious agents that passed through filters with a pore size small enough to trap bacteria. Then in the 1930s, the invention of the electron microscope allowed visualization of viruses and led to resolution of their structure and an understanding of their life cycle and recognition of the different families. Once it was realized that viruses are parasites that grow inside cells, cell culture techniques were developed for their propagation and isolation. These included growth in hens' eggs and in cultured cells, both of which showed a virus-induced cytopathic effect (CPE) on virus-infected cells which are characteristic of specific viruses. However, diagnosis based on hunting for a culprit virus by electron microscopy was extremely inefficient and time-consuming, while CPE formation in eggs or cultured cells took several days and was only successful with a proportion of pathogenic viruses. Thus until recently, the many virus infections were never diagnosed, and for those that were, the patient had usually recovered or died before the result came through. Indeed, with no specific treatment for virus infections in those days, many thought this did not matter.

The invention of monoclonal antibodies in the 1970s provided reagents specific for individual virus proteins that could be used to detect infected cells directly in diseased tissues. Also, antibodies to specific viruses could be detected in blood samples, and this became the mainstay of virus diagnosis until the recent molecular revolution. Rapid diagnosis can now be achieved by detection of tiny amounts of viral DNA or RNA in patient samples, so that there is little further need for virus culture or isolation. The breakthrough came with the invention of the polymerase chain reaction (PCR) in the 1980s. This technique has been adapted to detect and amplify specific viral genome sequences from clinical samples in minutes. Same-day diagnosis is now a reality, along with rapid assessments of viral loads and antiviral drug sensitivity.

While revolutionizing viral diagnosis, the PCR technique has also uncovered major diagnostic gaps. Diagnostic laboratories are still unable to find a culprit virus in many so-called 'viral' meningitis, encephalitis, and respiratory infections. This strongly suggests that there are many pathogenic viruses waiting to be discovered, and here too the PCR is a key research tool. With the human genome now fully sequenced, it is possible to identify 'foreign' genes in human clinical samples. Several 'new' viruses have recently been discovered in this way, including the human bocavirus, found to be a common cause of respiratory infections in children. But these discoveries are just the beginning; we can expect to hear about many more 'new' viruses over the next few years.

Chapter 9

Viruses past, present, and future

The study of viruses is less than 100 years old, but viruses themselves are ancient parasites whose history and evolution is closely entwined with our own.

Until the farming revolution began some 10,000 years ago, our ancestors were hunter-gatherers, living in small groups and constantly moving from place to place. The population was sparse, but still persistent viruses like the herpesviruses were able to thrive. They are clearly well adapted to the hunter-gatherer lifestyle, managing to infect almost everyone by biding their time until they could be passed on from one generation to the next. These viruses probably posed little threat, but with the change to the more settled farming lifestyle came the problem of zoonoses. The many 'new' viruses that jumped from domestic animals to the early farmers caused severe infections. By killing off the most susceptible in the population, these microbes have influenced our social history.

Smallpox virus in particular has killed untold millions since it transferred from its animal source, an event that probably took place around 5,000 to 10,000 years ago in the early communities of the fertile Euphrates, Tigris, Nile, Ganges, and Indus river valleys where farming thrived. Certainly, ancient Egyptian texts written around 3730 BC refer to a smallpox-like disease, and some

Egyptian mummies, including that of King Ramses V dating from 1157 BC, have skin lesions resembling smallpox.

The first documented epidemic was the plague of Athens in 430 BC that occurred during the Peloponnesian War between the Athenians led by Pericles and the Spartans and is thought by most experts to have been caused by smallpox. When Pericles decided to enclose Athens against the advancing Spartan infantry, he was unknowingly providing microbes with an ideal environment to thrive. As the city became severely overcrowded with refugees fleeing the advancing Spartans, the virus took hold, raging for four years and killing thousands, including Pericles himself. This spelled doom for the Athenians, and their defeat heralded the end of the Greek Empire.

As the populations of cities in Europe and Asia grew, so smallpox became a regular visitor, killing up to 30% of those it infected. As testimony to its devastating effects, the Indian tribal goddess Shitala, the Chinese goddess T'ou-Shen Niang-Niang, and the Christian saint Nicaise are all dedicated to smallpox, prayed to by the masses in the hope of preventing, or being cured of, the infection. Although the virus tended to hit the poor in their crowded, airless dwellings, the royalty of Europe were also dealt a blow from time to time. In the 18th century, smallpox caused the demise of the House of Stuart in the UK (1603–1701) (see Box 3), with other royal victims of the time including Joseph I of Germany, Hungary, and Bohemia (1678–1711), Louis I of Spain (1707–24), Louis XV of France (1710–74), Ulrika Eleonora of Sweden (1688–1741), and Peter II of Russia (1715–30), all dying within an 80-year period.

Smallpox was unknown in the 'New World' until it was introduced, along with many other microbes, by the Spanish conquistadors in the 16th century. With no immunity or genetic resistance to the virus, Native Americans suffered severely. Whole tribes were wiped out, and the population dropped by 90% over

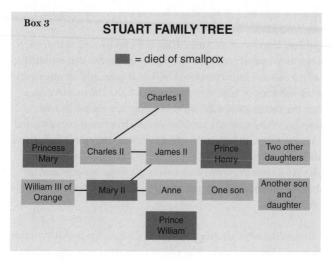

Box 3

STUART FAMILY TREE

■ = died of smallpox

Charles I

Princess Mary — Charles II — James II — Prince Henry — Two other daughters

William III of Orange — Mary II — Anne — One son — Another son and daughter

Prince William

the following 120 years. When the Spanish invaders arrived, the Aztecs in Mexico and the Incas in Peru each had a population of 20 to 30 million, with massive armies. Nevertheless, in 1521 Hernando Cortés defeated the Aztecs with around 600 soldiers, and Francisco Pizarro similarly conquered the Incas with just 200 men in 1532. Both men were aided by smallpox, possibly combined with other microbes, that concomitantly killed up to half the population, leaving the survivors so confused and demoralized that the Spanish invaders had easy victories.

Plant viruses have also had their moments of glory, and one such occurred during the 17th century when 'tulipmania' hit Holland. Tulips had recently been imported from Turkey and Dutch plant breeders were busy developing new varieties, including 'broken tulips' with white stripes on their flowers called 'colour breaks'. Owning such a plant became a status symbol in Holland, where

Viruses past, present, and future

between 1634 and 1637 a single bulb of the prized 'Admiral van Enkhuiijsen' variety could change hands for up to 5,400 guilders, the cost of an Amsterdam town house and 15 times a labourer's annual wage. But the plants were weak and unreliable; only occasional bulbs produced broken flowers and no one could work out why, or how to encourage the trait. The explanation is that the Dutch grew their bulbs in fields surrounded by fruit trees and virus-carrying aphids from the trees randomly dropped onto the tulips, infecting the plants, suppressing colour formation, and weakening the bulbs. Today, the multitude of variegated plants on offer at garden centres are also virus-infected and for that reason are generally not as vigorous as their plain-coloured counterparts.

Viruses, like other microbes, frequently use insects or other vectors to spread between hosts. The yellow fever virus uses mosquitoes to jump from one monkey to the next in the rain forests of West Africa. Infected monkeys remain healthy but if a virus-laden mosquito bites a human it causes a potentially deadly disease. This may be a flu-like illness, but in up to 20% of cases it progresses to a haemorrhagic fever with a high mortality. Humans often pick up the virus while felling trees in the jungle, an occupation that brings the infected mosquitoes down from the tree canopy into direct contact with the tree-fellers. Once humans are infected, the virus can be spread from person to person by urban mosquitoes, so causing an epidemic (Figure 19).

Yellow fever first appeared in the New World in the mid-17th century having hitched a ride aboard slave ships. Since the virus does not persist in those who recover from the infection, it must have survived the journey by infecting a series of victims on board, ferried between them by mosquitoes breeding in the ship's water barrels. Virus-carrying mosquitoes from the ships then moved inland and established an outpost in the Americas where they

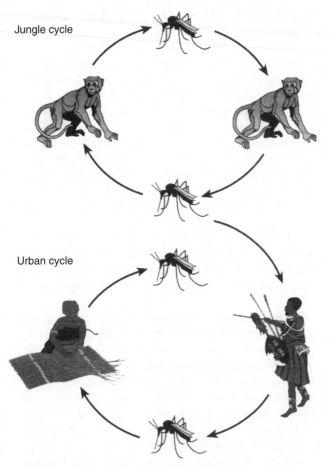

Jungle cycle

Urban cycle

19. The yellow fever transmission cycle, showing the jungle and urban cycles

remain today. Yellow fever caused devastating epidemics in both South and North America, killing thousands before the link with mosquitoes was unravelled in the late 19th century and preventive measures were taken.

Undoubtedly, yellow fever virus, along with smallpox, measles, malaria, and other imported microbes, had a hand in the depopulation of the Caribbean islands, attacking Native Americans, African slaves, and European settlers with equal ferocity. Indeed, Napoleon intended to make Santa Domingo the capital of his New World Empire and port of entry to the French property of Louisiana until yellow fever put a stop to his dreams. His army was unable to quell the slave rebellion led by Toussaint Louverture that began in 1791. Although he sent reinforcements, by 1802 his army had lost more than 40,000 troops, many to yellow fever. They were forced to surrender and quit the island, so ending Napoleon's hopes of expansion into the New World, and he sold the state of Louisiana to the US for 15 million dollars.

Yellow fever also defeated French attempts to build the Panama Canal in the late 19th century. They struggled for 20 years before giving up. The project was completed by the Americans in 1913 with a total death toll of 28,000 and a cost of 300 million dollars.

Small as they are, viruses still have the power to undermine our social structures today. From its small beginning in the rain forests of Cameroon around 100 years ago, HIV has caused the largest human pandemic in living memory. Over the last 50 years, it has ravaged sub-Saharan Africa, wiping out a generation of young people and depriving the next of family life and an education. The worst-hit countries have lost their valuable work force, plunging millions into poverty and accentuating the world's rich/poor divide. The HIV front has now moved to South-East Asia and Eastern Europe, where Russia has an estimated 1.5 million infected people. All along, governments' responses have largely been too little too late, and politicians appear powerless to stop its advance.

The HIV pandemic has seemed inexorable, but at last there are hopeful signs. International agencies working hand-in-hand with local organizations are turning the tide by delivering funding and aid, such as self-help programmes and the appropriate education to provide for their sustainability. The HIV pandemic is history-in-the-making; only time will tell what effect it has had on the world's social development.

What can we expect from viruses in the future?

We know that viruses are everywhere and that the virosphere is hugely diverse. This reservoir will certainly throw up new human pathogens from time to time; the question is: are we prepared? More specifically, can we predict, control, treat, and prevent new human virus infections? In Chapter 8, we saw how the genomic revolution impacted on virology, providing new, rapid diagnostic tests, targeted vaccines, and designer antiviral drugs. The outcome of the SARS epidemic in 2001 shows how these tools can be used effectively. As soon as the SARS coronavirus was identified, its genome was sequenced and diagnostic tests were prepared, all within a matter of months. The culprit animal source in Chinese wet markets was uncovered and now bats have been identified as the most likely long-term animal reservoir. Should the virus raise its ugly head again, we are ready with antiviral drugs and vaccines. A similar scenario, although on a much wider scale, occurred during the 2009 swine flu pandemic. The virus genome was rapidly sequenced, antivirals were made available for prevention and treatment, and a vaccine was prepared within six months. Even so, both SARS and swine flu had spread far beyond their point of origin before they were identified as a threat, indicating that prediction of an outbreak can be the weak link in the chain.

Although we know that most emerging viruses, including flu and SARS, jump from animals to humans, we are far from predicting when and where the next viral threat will appear. Indeed, in the case of flu, ever since the 1950s when WHO established the Global Influenza Surveillance Network involving over 90 countries, great efforts have been made to spot new flu strains that might cause the next pandemic. But still in 2009, when all attention was focused on the H5N1 bird flu in Asia, the emergence of H1N1 swine flu in Mexico went unnoticed. Clearly, studying and monitoring potentially threatening viruses in their primary animal host, like flu viruses in wild birds and retroviruses in primates, is a sensible way forward. But this would be a time-consuming and expensive occupation that few governments or agencies are prepared to fund. At present, all we can do is keep a sharp lookout for new clinical disease patterns that might indicate an emerging infection and nip it in the bud.

In parallel to hunting for emerging viruses, we can also search for viral causes of 'orphan' diseases. One such is chronic fatigue syndrome (CFS; previously called myalgia encephalomyelitis, or ME), which has long been recognized as a rather vague collection of symptoms. Recently, it has been defined as 'severe physical and mental fatigue without other clinical signs that is not relieved by rest and is of at least six months' duration'. The syndrome affects around 250,000 people in the UK and has now been recognized by the UK Department of Health as a debilitating, chronic disease. However, the cause of CFS is unknown; some favour a psychological origin while others suspect an infectious agent. Potential viral causes including enteroviruses, EBV, and other herpesviruses have hit the headlines from time to time, but so far the evidence is unconvincing. In 2009, researchers from the US examined over 100 CFS patients and reported finding a recently discovered mouse retrovirus called XMRV (or xenotropic murine leukaemia virus-related virus) in approximately two-thirds of patients. This suggested that antiretroviral therapy could benefit CSF sufferers, but unfortunately the findings could not be repeated by scientists in the UK. This could mean that CSF in the US and UK has different causes, but for now the debate as to whether CSF has an infectious or psychological origin continues.

In addition to predicting and identifying 'new' infections, we can also expect virus discovery to continue apace in the 21st century. Using modern molecular technologies, it is likely that many diseases, including some cancers, will be identified as viral, leading to preventive vaccines and novel treatments. A few therapeutic vaccines designed to boost the anti-tumour virus immune response in people who already have a virus-associated tumour are already in clinical trials. And as our knowledge of immune interactions increases, more sophisticated manipulation of the immune response should be feasible, tipping the balance in favour of tumour destruction. In this regard, immunotherapy trials using a variety of tools including specific antibodies and T cells to target virus-infected tumour cells are giving promising results, and the hope is that where appropriate this more natural form of treatment might replace chemotherapy and radiotherapy regimens with their unpleasant side effects.

Interestingly, there are indications that, in addition to causing traditional infectious diseases, viruses also play a role in the causation of certain non-infectious, chronic diseases. Multiple sclerosis (MS) is a debilitating disease of the nervous system which generally affects young adults and runs a chronic, relapsing course. Progressive nerve damage is caused by autoimmune destruction of the myelin sheath that surrounds nerve fibres, slowing and distorting the impulses they carry. The trigger for the production of autoantibodies directed against the myelin protein is unknown, although both inherited and environmental factors are implicated.

The epidemiology of MS and glandular fever caused by EBV is quite similar in that both are most common among high socioeconomic groups in affluent countries. This suggests that, like glandular fever, MS may be triggered by a delayed primary infection with an unknown virus. Indeed, MS is significantly more common in those who have suffered from glandular fever, and evidence is accumulating for a direct link between EBV and MS.

This is difficult to prove because almost everyone is infected with EBV but only a very small minority develop MS. However, recent studies show that whereas over 99% of adults with MS are infected with EBV, the level in matched, healthy control groups is around 90%. This means that an EBV-negative person is extremely unlikely to develop MS, but exactly why this should be, and whether EBV is causally linked to MS, remains unclear.

Another example is the herpesvirus cytomegalovirus (CMV), found as a persistent infection in approximately 50% of the developed world's population, which has been linked to coronary heart disease. The virus can be found in atheromatous plaques in diseased arteries where the chronic inflammation it causes may contribute to the subsequent blockage of blood flow that precipitates a heart attack. Another novel finding is that among the elderly, those with persistent CMV infection die earlier than those without. This is thought to be due to the long-term accumulation of CMV-specific immune T cells that in old age literally leave no room for an adequate immune response to other infectious agents.

These intriguing associations certainly warrant further investigation. As we have seen with cancer, although viruses may represent only one link in the chain of events that leads to a disease, their removal could prevent the disease occurring. These indirect effects of herpesviruses encourage some to think that several of our persistent viruses at present considered harmless may contribute to other common disorders.

During this century, we can look forward to man-made threats that in the worst-case scenario may impact on our burden of virus infections.

The idea of using microbes as weapons of mass destruction has been around for a long time, and the fact that it was prohibited by the Geneva Protocol of 1925 did not stop several countries running extensive programmes to develop and test the best candidates. Even the Biological Toxic Weapons convention of 1975 failed to halt this activity entirely, and nowadays the main threat is from terrorist groups.

The release of anthrax bacillus in the US in the aftermath of 9/11 certainly focused the world's attention on the threat posed by biological weapons, and some Western governments have since stockpiled the necessary drugs and vaccines to counteract such an attack. Although the rumours of biological weapons in Saddam Hussein's Iraq turned out to be false, in 2003's Operation Iraqi Freedom, troops went into battle vaccinated, wearing protective clothing, and swallowing antibiotics – thought by some to be the cause of 'Gulf War syndrome'.

Since they are relatively cheap and easy to prepare in factories masquerading as vaccine-production plants, the worry is that deadly microbes can be manufactured by terrorist groups. Their use would be difficult to detect in time to prevent a full-scale disaster as they are invisible, odourless, tasteless, often stable, effective in tiny quantities, and easily transportable across international frontiers without detection. They have the potential for targeted attacks, and broader application affecting large populations. Their delayed action allows the perpetrator time to escape. Several viruses feature in the list of potential threats, with Ebola and smallpox viruses being among the most deadly. Other viruses could be used to debilitate populations as opposed to killing them. Viruses such as rotavirus, causing diarrhoea and vomiting, could certainly weaken a population, but should be treatable.

Ebola virus poses a great threat, particularly in small communities, due to it being highly infectious, easily spread from person to person, with high mortality rates. But, as noted in Chapter 3, although explosive, Ebola outbreaks are usually self-limiting because of the necessity for direct spread: the short incubation period, and the devastating symptoms prevent sufferers from travelling far from the scene. Thus, as soon as the chain of infection is broken by barrier nursing, the outbreak can be controlled.

The situation would be entirely different with a virus like smallpox, phials of which are kept in two high-security laboratories, one in the US and the other in Russia. Some suspect that virus stocks may have been raided during political upheavals accompanying the break-up of the Soviet Union and could in theory have got into the hands of terrorist groups. The incubation period for smallpox is 12 to 24 days, which would enable worldwide dissemination before the first cases emerged. The virus, if released, could be devastating as it is easily spread, is stable, and requires just one or two particles to infect a person. This threat has led some governments to stockpile smallpox vaccine for just such an eventuality, but in reality it would be impossible to vaccinate a whole population in time to stop a pandemic. People vaccinated before the eradication campaign ended in 1977 may still be immune, but the majority of the world's population would be susceptible and the death rate likely to be around 30%.

Man-made virus threats are not restricted to the use of weapons of mass destruction, but include the unwitting promotion of pathogenic viruses. For example, xenotransplantation, the use of organs from animals such as pigs to replace diseased human organs in humans, may seem a sensible way to overcome the present waiting list for organs. But we know next to nothing about the viruses carried by these animals, and the little we do know about pig viruses suggests that their retroviruses can infect human cells. In addition, the success of several modern therapies, including transplantation and cancer chemotherapy, has resulted in an increasing number of people whose immune systems are suppressed. These people are more susceptible to virus infections, and in the absence of an adequate immune response viruses often persist long term. The worry is that immune-suppressed people could through no fault of their own become virus reservoirs, carrying and spreading unusual viruses in the community.

Laboratory escapees are also a cause for concern. Although mainly the subject of nightmares, virus escape is not unprecedented – note the flu virus that escaped from a Russian laboratory and caused a pandemic in 1977 (see Chapter 4), and the smallpox virus escape from a microbiology lab at Birmingham University, UK, in 1978 (see Chapter 8). With viruses now commonly used as vectors for foreign genes in the laboratory, extreme safety measures are warranted when handling this material. Genetically manipulated viruses are also being used in clinical trials to deliver a dose of vaccine or to correct a gene defect. In an early gene therapy trial, disaster struck when the retrovirus vector used to deliver a correcting gene to children with inherited immunodeficiency led to problems. Two out of 10 patients treated later developed leukaemia due to retroviral integration into their DNA close to a proto-oncogene called LMO2. These children's leukaemia was successfully treated, but still this incident was a severe setback for the clinical application of genetic manipulation. However, whereas few would suggest that this type of research, which has the potential to prevent, treat, and cure many diseases, should stop, most would agree it is right that it proceeds with caution.

Currently, we are in an exciting era of rapid technological advance somewhat akin to the Industrial Revolution of 19th-century Britain. This will certainly lead to vastly improved medical treatments, but we must ensure that our enthusiasm does not outstrip our ability to proceed safely. Therapeutic advances must always be informed by basic research that illuminates our understanding of disease processes.

We should heed the warning of virologist George Klein:

'The stupidest virus is cleverer than the cleverest virologist.'

Glossary

The words that are in italics in the Glossary entries indicate that these terms also appear as headwords, and so can be cross-referred to for a definition, rather than repeating the definitions at each entry.

aciclovir: a drug that inhibits the growth of certain *herpesviruses*. Used mostly to prevent or treat genital and oral herpes and shingles.

acquired immunodeficiency syndrome (AIDS): the stage of *human immunodeficiency virus* infection characterized by recurrent opportunistic infections.

acute retroviral syndrome: the syndrome caused by primary infection with *human immunodeficiency virus* characterized by malaise, fever, sore throat, enlarged glands, and a rash, lasting 2 to 6 weeks.

adenovirus: a DNA virus named after the human adenoid, from which it was first isolated. The virus causes respiratory and eye infections and has been used as a vector for DNA sequences in experimental gene therapy.

aflotoxin B1: a *toxin* produced by the mould *Apergillus flavis*.

antibody: a molecule made by *B lymphocytes* that circulates in the blood and body fluids and that can bind to and neutralize a specific *antigen*.

antigen: a foreign substance, usually a protein, that is capable of inducing an immune response in the body.

antigenic drift: the slow accumulation of *mutations* in the *genome* of a virus such as flu virus that eventually allows it to overcome the immune response generated against its parent virus.

antigenic shift: a major genetic change in a viral *genome*, such as a flu virus, resulting from gene reassortment and possibly generating a *pandemic* strain.

aphid: a small insect that feeds on plant sap.

apoptosis: controlled cell death. From the Greek 'apo' and 'ptosis' meaning 'falling off'. Also called programmed cell death.

Archaea: one of the three domains in the tree of life, the other two being Bacteria and Eukarya.

atheromatous plaque: a fatty deposit in the lining of an artery causing narrowing of the vessel and predisposing to blockage.

atypical pneumonia: inflammation of lung tissue induced by factors other than bacteria.

autoimmune disease: a disease caused by immune cells or *antibodies* reacting with and damaging normal body structures.

Bacillus anthracis: the bacterium that causes anthrax, so named because of the black colour of the lesions.

bacteriophage: a group of viruses that infect bacteria.

bacterium: a unicellular micro-organism in the domain Bacteria.

base pairs: the pairs of nucleotides that form the 'letters' of the genetic code. In *DNA*, adenine (A) pairs with thymine (T), and cytosine (C) pairs with guanine (G).

bluetongue virus: midge-borne virus of the Orbivirus genus, so called because of the orb-shaped *capsid*.

B lymphocyte/B cell: an *antibody*-producing cell that develops from stem cells in the bone marrow, circulates in the blood, and matures in lymph nodes.

bocavirus: a parvovirus, its name being derived from its two known hosts, cattle and dogs (i.e. **bo**vine and **ca**nine), recently identified as a cause of childhood respiratory disease in humans.

bronchiolitis: inflammation of the bronchioles – the smaller air passages of the lungs.

capsid: the protein coat surrounding the genetic material of a virus.

capsomere: a protein subunit of the viral *capsid*.

CD4: a molecule on the surface of *T cells* denoting their helper function.

CD8: a molecule on the surface of *T cells* denoting their cytotoxic (killer) function.

cervical intra-epithelial neoplasia (**CIN**): a precancerous condition of the uterine cervix that is confined to the surface epithelium.

chemokine receptor type 5 (**CCR5**): a cell surface molecule that acts as an essential co-receptor for HIV entry.

chromosome: a thread-like structure of *DNA* and protein that carries the *genes*. Found in the cell *nucleus*.

chromosome translocation: the transfer of genetic material incorrectly from one *chromosome* to another, causing a chromosome abnormality.

chronic fatigue syndrome (**CFS**): an illness characterized by severe fatigue of over 6 months' duration and without other clinical signs. Also called myalgia encephalomyelitis (ME).

cirrhosis: scarring of the liver caused by a *toxin* or virus and leading to liver failure.

c-myc: an *oncogene* implicated in several forms of cancer, including Burkitt's lymphoma.

co-evolution: linked evolution of two species, usually with mutual benefit to those species.

cold sore: a skin lesion, usually appearing on the face around the lips, caused by the herpes simplex virus.

conjunctivitis: inflammation of the surface epithelium (conjunctiva) of the eye.

croup: a harsh cough in children due to infection of the larynx and trachea, often by parainfluenza virus or *respiratory syncitial virus*.

cyanobacteria: free-living bacteria capable of photosynthesis. Previously known as blue-green algae.

cyanophage: a virus which infects *cyanobacteria*.

cytokine: a soluble chemical messenger that regulates immune responses.

cytokine storm: a massive and inappropriate release of *cytokines* following over-stimulation of the immune system.

cytomegalic inclusion disease: a congenital disease caused by intrauterine infection with cytomegalovirus. Symptoms in the infant may include growth retardation, deafness, poor blood clotting, and inflammation of the liver, lungs, heart, and brain.

cytopathetic effect: the cell damage caused by growing certain types of virus in cultured cells.

cytoplasm: the part of a cell surrounding the *nucleus* that contains the *organelles*.

cytotoxic T cell (killer T cell): a *T lymphocyte* with the ability to kill virus-infected cells. These cells generally bear the *CD8* marker.

dengue fever virus: a flavivirus that causes dengue fever, often referred to as 'breakbone fever' because of the severe pains in the bones, joints, and muscles.

Devonian period: geological period spanning 416 to 359 million years ago; part of the Paleozoic Era. The name is derived from the county of Devon, where rocks of this period were first studied.

DNA (deoxyribonucleic acid): a self-replicating molecule that carries the genetic material in all organisms except *RNA* viruses.

Ebola virus: a filovirus (from the Latin *filum*, meaning thread and referring to the filamentous structure of these viruses) that causes Ebola haemorrhagic fever. Named after the Ebola River in Zaire near Yambuku, where the first reported outbreak occurred.

echovirus: **e**nteric **c**ytopathic **h**uman **o**rphan virus, a picornavirus (*pico* meaning small, *RNA* virus) so named because when it was first isolated, it was not associated with any disease. Now known to cause *conjunctivitis* and a flu-like febrile illness.

ecosystem: a self-sustaining community of interacting organisms.

electron microscope: a microscope that uses a beam of electrons instead of light. Magnifies over a hundred thousand times.

encephalitis: inflammation of the brain.

endemic: found regularly in a particular geographical area or population.

engraftment: inoculation with smallpox 'scabs' to induce immunity without severe disease. Also called variation.

epidemic: a large-scale temporary increase in a disease in a community or region.

Epstein–Barr virus (EBV): a virus which causes glandular fever (infectious mononucleosis) and is associated with a number of human tumours. The virus is named after the scientists who discovered it, Anthony Epstein and Yvonne Barr.

eukaryote: a member of the Eukarya domain, which includes all living things except Bacteria and Archaea.

evolutionary tree: see *phylogenetic tree*.

extremophile: a class of single-cell organisms able to survive in extreme environmental conditions.

Fertile Crescent: the geographical region in modern-day Iraq and Iran between the rivers Euphrates and Tigris where archaeologists think farming started.

filterable agent: the original term for a virus – an infectious agent that passes through a filter with a pore size small enough to retain a bacterium.

flavivirus: a family of insect-borne viruses that includes the yellow fever virus, the name being derived from the Latin *flavus* for yellow.

flu virus: see *influenza virus*.

gene: the part of a *chromosome*, usually *DNA*, which codes for a specific protein.

gene deregulation: loss of control of expression of a specific *gene*.

genetic material: see *DNA* and *RNA*.

genome: the *genetic material* of an organism.

glandular fever: see *Epstein–Barr virus (EBV)*.

Gonococcus: known also as *Neisseria gonorrhoeae*, a sexually transmitted bacterium.

Gulf War syndrome: a variable combination of psychological and physical symptoms experienced by Gulf War veterans.

haemaglutinin: an *influenza virus* surface protein that acts as a virus receptor and induces an immune response.

helper T cell: a *T lymphocyte* that bears the *CD4* marker and helps other lymphocyte subsets generate an immune response.

Hendra virus: a paramyxovirus originally called equine morbillivirus. Named after the place of Hendra, in Australia, where it caused an outbreak of fatal respiratory infection in horses and humans in 1994.

hepatitis B virus: a major cause of chronic liver disease and liver cancer. A *DNA* virus in the hepadnavirus family, this name deriving from *hepa* (i.e. liver), DNA, and virus.

herpesvirus: a family of *DNA* viruses including those causing *cold sores*, chickenpox, and shingles. The name 'herpes' is derived from the Greek *herpeton*, meaning reptile, and probably refers to the creeping nature of the lesions of shingles.

highly active antiretroviral therapy (**HAART**): combination drug therapy used to treat *HIV* infection.

human immunodeficiency viruses (**HIVs**): a group of *retroviruses* that cause AIDS. To date, humans have been infected with HIV-1 strains M, N, O, P, and HIV-2, all of which were acquired from African primates.

hygiene hypothesis: the theory that a lack of exposure to infectious agents during childhood predisposes to allergic and autoimmune diseases.

immunological memory: the ability of the immune system to 'remember' previous exposure to an infectious organism and prevent further attacks. Mediated by *memory T cells*.

immunopathology: tissue damage caused by the immune response.

incubation period: the period of time between infection and the onset of symptoms.

index case: the first case of an infectious disease in a population from which all others are derived.

influenza virus (**flu virus**): an orthomyxovirus that causes flu epidemics and pandemics. The disease was named 'influenza' (Italian for 'influence') in the 15th century, when it was believed that flu was caused by a malevolent supernatural influence.

inoculation: originally, a term that was used for the technique of infecting with a small dose of smallpox to induce immunity without severe disease. Now, it is used to mean injection with any infectious material.

integrase: the enzyme that facilitates *integration* of the retroviral *provirus* into host *DNA*.

integration: the process of incorporation of a *DNA* sequence into another DNA chain. This is an essential step in the *retrovirus* life cycle.

interferon: a family of *cytokines* with antiviral properties.

interleukin 2: a *cytokine* essential for *T cell* growth and survival.

jaundice: the yellow colouration of the skin and conjunctiva associated with liver disease.

JC virus: a polyomavirus that causes degenerative brain disease. Named after the initials of the patient from whom it was first isolated.

Kaposi sarcoma herpesvirus (KSHV): a *herpesvirus* (also called human herpesvirus 8, HHV 8) that causes Kaposi sarcoma, a condition named after the physician who first described the tumour.

killer T cell: see *cytotoxic T cell*.

Langerhans cell: a *macrophage* found in skin and on other body surfaces.

last universal cellular ancestor (LUCA): the common ancestor of the three domains of life: Archaea, Bacteria, and Eukaryota.

latent infection: a virus infection of a cell in which few or no viral proteins are expressed. Typical of a *herpesvirus* infection, allowing long-term persistence.

live attenuated vaccine: a *vaccine* preparation containing a non-pathogenic form of a microbe that induces immunity without disease.

lymphocytes: white blood cells with a variety of functional subsets that orchestrate the specific immune response (see *B*, *T*, *helper*, *cytotoxic*, *memory*, and *regulatory* T cells).

lytic phage: *bacteriophage* that infect and kill bacteria.

macrophage: a mobile immune cell found in the tissues where it initiates an immune response by production of *cytokines*. Macrophages engulf and destroy foreign and dead material, the name meaning 'large appetite'.

Marek's disease virus: a *herpesvirus* that causes tumours in chickens. Named after Jozef Marek who described the disease in 1907.

memory T cell: a long-lived *B* or *T lymphocyte* that has been stimulated by its specific *antigen* and can respond rapidly on a second encounter.

meningitis: inflammation of the meninges, the membranes surrounding the brain.

mesothelioma: a tumour of the mesothelial cells lining the lung cavity associated with inhalation of asbestos.

methicillin-resistant *Staphylococcus aureus* (MSRA): a bacterium that is resistant to most commonly used antibiotics. A problem in hospital infections.

microbe: the general term used to cover all microscopic organisms including viruses, bacteria, archaea, and the unicellular parasites.

mimivirus: a recently discovered virus which is so large that it was at first thought to be a bacterium. The name is derived from 'microbe-mimicking virus'.

mitochondria: cellular *organelles* responsible for respiration and the generation of energy. Thought to be derived from proteobacteria.

molecular clock: a measurement of the molecular difference between two *genomes* as a way of assessing the evolutionary distance between them.

monoclonal antibodies: monospecific *antibodies* made from a culture of cloned *B lymphocytes*. Used as reagents for identifying virus infections and for immunotherapy.

monocyte: a circulating immune cell that matures into a tissue *macrophage*.

mutation: a genetic change that is transmitted to offspring, giving inheritable variation.

Myalgia encephalomyelitis (ME): see *chronic fatigue syndrome*.

naked DNA vaccine: a *vaccine* composed of a *DNA* sequence coding for an immunogenic protein.

neoplasia: another name for a tumour or cancer, meaning 'new growth'.

neurominidase: an enzyme on the surface of *influenza virus* particles that destroys neuraminic (sialic) acid. It is part of the flu virus receptor for binding to cells and induces an immune response in infected hosts.

Nipah virus: a paramyxovirus related to *Hendra virus*. A natural infection of fruit bats, it can cause disease in other animals including *encephalitis* in humans. Named after the village in Malaysia where the person from whom it was first isolated lived.

norovirus: a calicivirus that causes outbreaks of acute gastroenteritis. Previously called Norwalk agent after an outbreak in the town of this name in the USA, the name was shortened to norovirus in 2002.

nosocomial infection: a hospital-acquired infection. Derived from the Greek word *nosokomeion*, meaning hospital.

nucleoside: a base, for example cytosine, bound to a sugar molecule. Nucleosides may be phosphorylated in a cell to form nucleotides, the building blocks of *DNA* and *RNA*.

nucleus: derived from *nuculeus*, the Latin word for kernel, it is a membrane-bound *organelle* that contains the *chromosomes* in *eukaryotic* cells.

obligate parasite: an organism, like a virus, that is entirely dependent on other life forms.

oncogene: a *gene* that can transform a normal cell into a tumour cell.

opportunistic infection: an infection that takes hold because the host is immunosuppressed.

orchitis: inflammation of the testis.

organelle: a subcellular structure such as a *nucleus*, *mitochondrium*, or *ribosome*.

Oseltamivir (Tamiflu): an antiviral drug active against the *influenza virus*. The drug blocks the activity of the viral neuraminidase enzyme, thereby preventing new viruses being released from infected cells.

pandemic: an *epidemic* involving more than one continent at once.

panspermia: the theory that life exists throughout the Universe and that microbes have been seeded to Earth via comets. The word is derived from the Greek *pan*, meaning all, and *spermia*, meaning seed.

papillomavirus: a family of viruses that cause benign epithelial tumours such as warts and verrucae, and malignant tumours of the uterine cervix, penis, and head and neck. The name derives from the Latin *papilla*, meaning nipple.

parasite: an organism living on or in another and benefiting at its expense.

parotid glands: bilateral glands in the cheek that produce saliva. Typically inflamed during mumps.

pathogen: an organism that causes disease.

photosynthesis: the chemical process that converts carbon dioxide into sugar and oxygen using solar energy. Principally carried out by plants.

phylogenetic tree (**evolutionary tree**): a branching diagram indicating the evolutionary relationship between different species.

phytoplankton: microscopic plants in the ocean that are at the bottom of the ocean's food chain.

plankton: the microscopic life forms that drift in the oceans.

plasmodesmata: microscopic channels in the cell walls of plants that allow molecular transport between adjacent cells.

pneumonia: inflammation of the lung tissue.

polymerase chain reaction (**PCR**): a technique for amplifying a single *DNA* sequence thousands or millions of times.

polymorph (**polymorphonuclear leucocyte**): a type of white blood cell named because of the varying shape of its lobed nucleus. Also may be called a granulocyte. Part of the immune attack against bacterial infections, these cells have granules that contain antimicrobial substances. They are attracted to sites of infection and die there, forming the substance of pus.

post-exposure vaccine: a *vaccine* given after infection in an attempt to prevent or ameliorate symptoms.

primary infection: the illness caused by an organism the first time it infects an individual. Characterized by an immunoglobulin M *antibody* response.

primordial soup: the mixture of naturally occurring chemicals from which life first arose.

programmed cell death: see *apoptosis*.

prokaryote: a group of organisms, including all bacteria and archaea, which do not have a *nucleus* or *organelles* and are usually unicellular.

proto-oncogene: an *oncogene* in a cellular *genome* that has been *transduced* by a virus.

provirus: virus sequences *integrated* into the host *genome*.

quasispecies: a group of closely related viruses that are *mutating* rapidly while competing with each other for *viral fitness*.

reactivation: the re-establishment of virus replication from a *latent infection*.

recombinant vaccine: a synthetic *vaccine* made from a subunit of a virus. May be a protein or *genome* sequence.

regulatory T cell: a *T cell* that controls the extent of the immune response by producing inhibitory *cytokines*.

respiratory syncitial virus: a cause of respiratory disease in children. So called because infection causes cell membranes to merge, forming syncitia.

retrovirus: a family of viruses that contains the *HIVs*. So called because they can reverse transcribe the *RNA* to *DNA* and *integrate* into the host *genome*.

reverse transcriptase: the enzyme used by *retroviruses* to reverse transcribe their *RNA genome* into *DNA*.

rhinovirus: the common cold virus. A picornavirus, the name derives from the Greek *rhis*, meaning nose.

ribosome: a cellular *organelle* that makes proteins from amino acids.

Rinderpest virus: a morbillivirus related to the measles virus. The name is German for 'cattle plague', the fatal disease of ruminants caused by the virus, now eliminated globally.

RNA (ribonucleic acid): one of the two types of nucleic acid that exist in nature, the other being *DNA*. It forms the genetic material of some viruses.

RNA interference: a system which controls *gene* expression by the binding of small complementary (interfering) *RNA* molecules to RNA strands. Also called gene silencing, this mechanism is used in defence against *microbes* and parasites.

rotavirus: a group of viruses that cause gastroenteritis in infants. The name derives from the Latin *rota*, meaning wheel, and denotes their wheel-like structure.

sacral ganglia: part of a chain of nerve ganglia, or nerve cell bodies, lying alongside the spinal cord in the sacral region.

SARS coronavirus: the cause of *SARS*. The coronavirus family are so called because of their crown-like structure.

severe acute respiratory syndrome (SARS): an emerging infection consisting of an acute respiratory illness that is fatal in around 10% of cases.

smallpox: a severe acute infection caused by the virus *Variola major*. Characterized by skin pocks and so called to distinguish the disease from the 'great pox' – syphilis.

squamous epithelium: the multilayered structure that covers the outer body, forming the skin and certain inner surfaces including the mouth, throat, oesophagus, and vagina.

subacute sclerosing pan encephalitis (SSPE): a rare, fatal consequence of measles caused by a persistent virus infection of brain tissue.

syphilis: a sexually transmitted disease caused by the bacterium *Treponema pallidum*.

Tamiflu: see *Oseltamivir*.

T cell (lymphocyte): the type of *lymphocyte* that generates the specific, cell-mediated immune response essential for control of virus infections. See also *helper, cytotoxic* (killer), *memory,* and *regulatory* T cells.

thymidine kinase: an enzyme found in most mammalian cells that phosphorylates deoxythymidine, an essential process for building *DNA*. Some viruses code for a viral thymidine kinase, a requirement for the action of certain antiviral drugs such as *aciclovir*.

tobacco mosaic virus: a tobamovirus (from **toba**cco **mo**saic) so called because of the mottled pattern it produces on the leaves of infected plants.

toxin: a soluble chemical poison produced by bacteria that can be destroyed by heat.

toxogenic phage: phage that contain a *toxin* gene and kill the bacteria they infect.

transduction: the acquisition of a cellular *gene* by a virus.

transformation: the alteration of a normal cell to a malignant cell.

Treponema pallidum: the spirochete bacterium that causes syphilis.

trigeminal ganglia: the bilateral nerve ganglia of the fifth cranial nerve situated at the base of the skull.

TT virus: a recently described, ubiquitous anellovirus. Named after the initials of the person from whom it was first isolated, it appears to be non-pathogenic.

tumour suppressor gene: a *gene* that negatively controls cell division. Several tumour viruses inactivate these genes, causing increased cell proliferation.

vaccination: the process of administering a *vaccine*. Derived from the Latin *vacca*, meaning cow, the word was originally applied to *smallpox* vaccination but is now used more widely.

vaccine: material derived from an infectious organism introduced into the body to generate a protective immune response without disease.

variolation: see *engraftment*.

vector: the means of viral transport from one host to another, for example via an insect. The term is also used for the artificial transfer of genetic material into cells or organisms, for example an adenovirus vector used to deliver 'foreign' *DNA* as a *vaccine*.

verruca: a plantar wart.

Vibrio cholerae: the bacterium that causes cholera.

viraemia: virus in the blood.

viral envelope: the loose membrane that surrounds some viruses, derived from cellular material.

viral fitness: the ability of a virus to compete with other strains of the same virus group.

viral load: a measurement of the level of a virus in the blood.

viral set point: the stable level of virus in the blood during a *latent* or persistent infection.

virion: a virus particle.

virosphere: the massive community of viruses in the environment.

virulence: the degree of pathogenicity of a *microbe* as indicated by its ability to invade, damage the tissues, and kill the host.

virus: a small infectious agent that can only replicate inside a living cell. The term 'virus' derives from the Latin, meaning a poison or noxious substance.

wart: a benign tumour of the skin caused by a *papillomavirus*.

Glossary

yellow fever virus: a mosquito-transmitted *flavivirus* that causes yellow fever, characterized by fever and *jaundice*.

zoonosis: an infectious disease of humans acquired from an animal source.

zoonotic virus: a virus that has jumped to humans from an animal host.

zooplankton: the invertebrate animal portion of *plankton*.

Further reading

Chapter 1

D. H. Crawford, *The Invisible Enemy: A Natural History of Viruses* (Oxford University Press, 2000).

Chapter 2

B. La Scola, S. Audic, C. Robert, L. Jungang, X. De Lamballerie, M. Drancourt, R. Birtles, J. M. Claverie, and D. Raoult, 'A Giant Virus in Amoebae', *Science*, 299 (2003): 2033.

C. A. Suttle, 'Viruses in the Sea', *Nature*, 437 (2005): 356–61.

L. Ledford, 'Death and Life Beneath the Sea Floor', *Nature*, 545 (2008): 1038.

K. M. Oliver, P. H. Degnan, M. S. Hunter, and N. A. Moran, 'Bacteriophages Encode Factors Required for Protection in a Symbiotic Mutualism', *Science*, 325 (2009): 992–4.

Chapter 3

P. Horvath and R. Barrangou, 'CRISPR/Cas, the Immune System of Bacteria and Archaea', *Science*, 327 (2010): 167–70.

Chapter 4

A. J. McMichael, 'Environmental and Social Influences on Emerging Infectious Diseases: Past, Present and Future', *Philosophical Transactions of the Royal Society, London* B 359 (2004): 1049–58.

M. E. J. Woolhouse, 'Population Biology of Emerging and Re-emerging Pathogens', *Trends in Microbiology*, 10 (Suppl., 2002): S3–S7.

Chapter 5

J. Diamond, *Guns, Germs and Steel: A Short History of Everybody for the Last 13,000 Years* (Vintage, 1998).

P. Aaby, 'Is Susceptibility to Severe Infection in Low-Income Countries Inherited or Acquired?', *Journal of Internal Medicine*, 261 (2007): 112–22.

P. Sharp and B. H. Hahn, 'The Evolution of HIV-1 and the Origin of AIDS', *Philosophical Transactions of the Royal Society, London* B, 2010.

J. F. Fears, 'The Plague under Marcus Aurelius and the Decline and Fall of the Roman Empire', *Infectious Disease Clinics of North America*, 18 (2004): 65–77.

Chapter 6

D. A. Thorley-Lawson, 'Epstein–Barr Virus: Exploiting the Immune System', *Nature Reviews Immunology*, 1 (2001): 75–82.

Chapter 7

E. D. Pleasance et al., 'A Comprehensive Catalogue of Somatic Mutations from a Human Cancer Genome', *Nature*, 463 (2010): 191–6.

A. S. Evans and N. E. Mueller, 'Viruses and Cancer: Causal Associations', *Annals of Epidemiology*, 1 (1990): 71–92.

Chapter 8

F. Fenner, D. A. Henderson, I. Arita et al., *Smallpox and Its Eradication* (WHO, Geneva, 1988).

A. J. Wakefield, S. H. Murch, A. Anthony et al., 'Ileal-Lymphoid-Nodular Hyperplasia, Non-Specific Colitis, and Pervasive Development Disorder in Children', *Lancet*, 351 (1998): 637–41.

C. Dyer, 'Lancet Retracts MMR Paper after GMC Finds Andrew Wakefield Guilty of Dishonesty', *British Medical Journal*, 349 (2010): 281.

A. S. Fauci, 'Pathogenesis of HIV Disease: Opportunities for New Preventive Interventions', *Clinical Infectious Diseases*, 45 (Suppl. 4, 2007): S206–12.

Chapter 9

D. H. Crawford, *Deadly Companions: How Microbes Shaped Our History* (Oxford University Press, 2007).

V. C. Lombardi et al., 'Detection of an Infectious Retrovirus, XMRV, in Blood Cells of Patients with Chronic Fatigue Syndrome', *Science*, 326 (2009): 585–9.

O. Erlwein et al., 'Failure to Detect the Novel Retrovirus XMRV in Chronic Fatigue Syndrome', *PLoS ONE*, 5 (2010): e8519.

S. Hacein-bey-Abina et al., 'LMO2-associated Clonal T Cell Proliferation in Two Patients after Gene Therapy for SCID-X1', *Science*, 302 (2003): 415–19.

Publisher's acknowledgements

Index

A

aciclovir 71, 115
AIDS 16, 36, 38–9, 43, 73–7, 93–4,
    112–13, 115 *see also* HIV
air travel 48
airborne viruses 2, 38, 52–94
antibodies 31–3, 61–2, 76, 80, 113,
    118, 127
antigens 30–1, 40–1, 78, 110, 112
antiretroviral drugs 12, 38, 77,
    114–16, 126
antiviral agents 12, 71, 76, 80, 82,
    114–18, 125
aphids 22, 27, 122
apoptosis 10
archaea 13, 16–19, 28–9

B

cells (lymphocytes) 31–2, 72, 91,
    93, 95
bacteria 2–4, 6–7, 13–14, 16–23,
    28–9, 63, 114–15, 117
Bang, Oluf 83
barrier nursing 38, 44, 64, 130
bats 43–5, 107, 125
Beijerinck, Martinus 3
Belloc, Hilaire 1–2
biological weapons 128–30

bird flu (H5N1) 34, 40–2, 126
blood and blood products 26–8
    coronary heart disease 128
    diagnosis 118
    hepatitis 28, 78, 81–2
    herpesviruses 91
    HIV 38–9, 74–7, 113–14
    leukaemia 88, 90
    placenta, transmission through
        the 31, 56, 71
bluetongue virus 47
breast-feeding 31, 38, 69,
    88, 90
bronchiolitis 57
Burkitt, Denis 91–1

C

cancer 35, 63, 66, 72, 76, 78,
    81–101, 112, 127–8, 130
capsids 4, 8, 15
CCR5 29, 40
CD4 T-cells 8, 31, 33, 40,
    74–6, 113
CD8 T-cells 31
cell culture 83–4, 86–8, 92, 96–8,
    108, 117–18
cervical cancer 86, 98–100, 112
chickenpox (*Varicella zoster virus*)
    51, 53, 56–7, 68, 70–1

childhood infections 51–62, 69–70, 72, 81, 91–2, 94, 109
cholera 2, 22–3
chronic fatigue syndrome (myalgia encephalomyelitis) 126
cirrhosis 78, 80–1, 95–6
Clostridium difficile 63
cold sores (herpes simplex) 27, 68–70, 76, 115
common cold (rhinovirus) 26–7, 53, 57–8, 108
conjunctivitis 57
coronary heart disease 128
cowpox 52, 103–5, 107
croup 57–8
cytokines 30–2, 42, 80, 117
cytomegalovirus (CMV) 68, 71, 128

D

de Maton, George 56
death rates
    AIDS/HIV 36, 38, 74
    cancer 84, 99
    flu 42
    hepatitis 116
    measles 55–6, 64
    rabies 108
    respiratory viruses 57–8
    Rinderpest 62
    rotaviruses 59
    SARS 36–8
    smallpox 103–5, 110–11, 120–1, 130
definition of virus 4
defences to viruses 28–33, 65
dengue fever 27, 45–7
diabetes 32
diagnosis 117–18, 125
DNA 2, 4, 7–15, 19, 33, 40, 65, 67, 74, 81, 86, 96–101, 106, 112, 115, 118, 131
drugs 12, 38, 70, 76–7, 82, 93, 114–18, 125, 129

E

Ebola and Ebola-like viruses 44, 63, 109, 129–30
electron microscopes 4, 14, 117–18
elimination or eradication of viruses 54–6, 62, 102–11, 130
Ellerman, Wilhelm 83
emerging virus infections 34–50, 125–7
Emiliania huxleyi 19
encephalitis 44–5, 49, 56, 66, 71, 78, 118
enteroviruses 61, 126
epidemics 35–7, 40–1, 44, 51–60, 103–5, 108, 111, 116, 120, 123
Epstein-Barr virus 27, 32, 66, 68, 72, 77, 91–4, 127–8
eukaryotes 13, 17–19
evolution 11–15, 17–19, 23, 29, 66–7, 80, 119

F

faecal-oral transmission 52–3, 59–64, 78, 109
farming revolution 51–2, 119
fighting viruses 25–33
flesh-eating bug (*Streptococcus pyogenes*) 63
flu 3, 18, 26, 32, 34, 40–2, 48, 51, 53, 58, 115–17, 125–6, 131
foot and mouth disease 48–9
future of viruses 125–31

G

Gallo, Robert 87
gastroenteritis 59–60, 62
genetic material or *genome* 4–20, 41, 60, 76, 84–7, 91, 94–8, 131
    see also DNA; RNA
genital herpes 68, 69–70
German measles (rubella) 3, 54, 56–7, 108, 110

glandular fever (kissing disease) 27, 68, 71–2, 127–8
Global Influenza Surveillance Network 125–6
gods 54, 120
Gregg, Norman 56
Gulf War syndrome 129
gut, viruses in the 21–2, 26–7, 30, 52–3, 59–64

H

Hamiltonella defensa 22
healthcare workers 28, 36–7, 114
Hendra virus 45
hepatitis A (HAV) 15, 78, 95
hepatitis B (HBV) 15, 27–8, 31, 66, 78–9, 81–2, 95–6, 110, 112, 116–17
hepatitis C (HCV) 15, 31, 66, 78–81, 95–7, 116–17
hepatitis D (HDV) 78, 95
hepatitis E (HEV) 78, 95
hepatitis viruses 15, 27–8, 31, 66, 77–82, 95–7, 110, 112, 116–17
herpesviruses 4, 6, 27, 66–72, 76, 77, 90–5, 100, 115, 119, 126, 128
HIV
    antiviral drugs 114–16
    antiretroviral drugs 12, 38, 114–15
    blood and blood products 38–9, 74–7, 113–14
    central nervous system 76–7
    death rates 38, 74
    immune system 8–12, 29, 33, 39, 71, 73, 76, 93, 113
    Kaposi sarcoma-associated virus (KSHV) 66, 68, 72, 91, 94–5
    mutations 13, 33
    non-sexual transmission routes 38–9
    origins 39, 43, 73
    receptors 8
    resistance 29
    sexual transmission 27–8, 38–9, 74

stages 74–5
tumour viruses 93–4
vaccinations 112–14
worldwide effects 124–5
Hodgkin's lymphoma 94
Hoffman, Friedrich 56
hospital-acquired or nosocomial infections 62–4
Hoyle, Fred 23
hygiene 26, 48, 52–3, 61–2, 78, 110

I

immune systems 28–33, 64–6, 70–6
    avoiding immune attacks, viruses 25–6, 28–33, 86
    common cold 57
    hepatitis 117
    HIV 8–12, 29, 33, 39, 71, 73, 76, 93, 113
    immunopathology 32, 80
    reservoirs, immuno-suppressed people as 130–1
    tumour viruses 86, 91, 93–4, 127
    vaccinations 110
immunity 28, 33, 40–2, 51, 54, 60, 64–7, 70, 76, 80, 102–3
incubation period 35–8, 54, 57, 59, 63, 90, 106, 130
insects 8, 22, 26, 28, 45–7, 49, 122–3
isolation of microbes 1–3
Ivanovsky, Dmitry 3

J

Jenner, Edward 102–4, 107, 110
Jesty, Benjamin 103–4

K

Kaposi sarcoma-associated virus (KSHV) 66, 68, 72, 91, 94–5, 101
Koch, Robert 2

Index

L

laboratory animals 83–5
laboratory escapes 131
last universal cellular ancestor (LUCA) 13–14
latent infections 67–9
leukaemia 66, 83, 87–90, 131
liver damage 77–8, 80–1, 95–6, 116
lymphocytes 8, 30–3, 39–40, 54, 66, 72, 74–6, 80, 87, 93–4, 107, 113, 128

M

Maitland, Charles 103
malaria 44, 55, 93, 114, 124
Marek's disease 107
marine environment 17–23
Mayer, Adolf 3
measles 3, 12–13, 26 , 52–7, 62, 63–4, 110–11, 124
Medawar, Peter 4
meningitis 59, 61, 118
methicillin-resistant
    Staphylococcus pyogenes
    (MRSA) 63
microbes 1–4, 16–19, 21–3, 27–34, 45, 50–2, 66, 119–22, 128–9
microscopes 2, 4, 14, 117–18
mimivirus (microbe-mimicking virus) 4, 6, 8, 17–18
MMR (measles, mumps and rubella) vaccine 56
molecular clock hypothesis 12–13, 52
Montague, Mary Wortley 102–4
Moore, Patrick 94, 101
mortality rates *see* death rates
mosquitoes 27, 45, 49, 122–3
MRSA (methicillin-resistant
    Staphylococcus pyogenes) 63
multiple sclerosis 32, 72, 127–8
mumps 3, 53–4, 56–7, 110, 124
mutations 10–13, 29, 31, 33, 40–2, 60, 65, 76, 80, 84–7, 93–4, 106

myalgia encephalomyelitis (chronic fatigue syndrome) 126

N

New World 88, 120–4
Nipah virus 45
nosocomial infections 62–4
noroviruses 26, 59–61, 63
nucleotides 11

O

oceans 17–23
oncogenes 84, 86–7, 91, 93–5, 99–100
outer space 22–3
overpopulation 48–9

P

pandemics 34–42, 53–4, 73, 116, 124–6, 130–1
panspermia 23
papilloma viruses 18, 66, 27, 97–100
parasites 13–14, 23, 82, 117, 119
past, viruses in the 2–4, 14–15, 38–63, 66, 83–8, 91–2, 102–24
Pasteur, Louis 2, 107–8
Peloponnesian War 120
penicillin 114–15
persistent viruses 65–82, 116–17
phages 16–17, 19–23, 26, 28–30, 66, 71, 74
photosynthesis 19–21
phytoplankton 19–21
placenta 31, 56, 71
plankton 19–21
pneumonia 17, 36–7, 53, 55, 57–9, 71, 76
polio 61–2, 108–10
polymerase chain reaction (PCR) 118
poverty 38, 48, 74, 120, 124
pox viruses 3–4, 6, 9, 13, 52 *see also* cowpox; smallpox

protein 2, 4, 6, 8–9, 13–14, 18, 20, 28–30, 32, 67, 111–12, 127
provirus 9–10, 33

R

rabies 4, 107–8, 110
receptors 8, 30–1, 78
recombinant vaccines 111–13
regulatory T cells 32, 80
reproduction 8–14, 20–1, 25–6
retroviruses 9–10, 12, 14, 66, 72–7, 86–8, 91, 130 see also AIDs; HIV
reverse transcriptase (RT) 9, 14, 87–8
rheumatoid arthritis 72
rhinovirus (common cold) 26–7, 53, 57–8, 108
Rinderpest virus 52, 62
rise in infections 38, 45, 47–50
RNA 4–5, 8–12, 14–15, 28–9, 41, 78, 80, 95, 118
RNAi (RNA interference) 28–9
rotaviruses 26–7, 59–60, 62, 129
Rous, Peyton 83–4, 97
royalty affected by smallpox 120–1
rubella (German measles) 3, 54, 56–7, 108, 110

S

Sabin, Albert 100
Salk, Jonas 109
SARS coronavirus 16, 34–8, 40, 43–4, 48, 63, 125
sexual transmission 27–8, 38–9, 69, 74, 81, 91, 98–9
shape of viruses 4, 14–15, 17
shingles 57, 70–1
Shope, Richard 97
silent infections 37–9, 61, 63, 66, 69–73, 77, 81, 90, 95, 106
size of viruses 4, 6, 14, 17, 21
smallpox 3, 13, 29, 52–3, 102–7, 110–11, 119–21, 124, 129–30

squamous epithelial cells 97–9
structure of viruses 4, 5, 15, 17, 117
subacute sclerosing pan
    encephalitis (SSPE) 66
swine flu (H1N1) 34, 41–2, 48, 116, 125–6
syphilis 2, 28

T

Takatsuki, Kiyoshi 87–8
Tamiflu 116
T-cells 8, 31–3, 39–40, 66, 72, 74–6, 80, 87–90, 93–4, 107, 113, 127–8
terrorism 129
tobacco mosaic disease 3–4
tropical spastic paraparesis (non-malignant myelopathy) 87
TTV 65–6
tuberculosis 2, 18, 76
tulipmania 121–2
tumour viruses 35, 66, 72, 76, 78, 81–101, 127–8, 131
turtle papillomavirus 18

V

vaccinations 12, 33, 54–7, 61–4, 80–2, 96, 99–114, 125
van Leeuwenhoek, Antonie 2
Vibrio cholerae 22
viral shunt 20–1
virosphere 15–24, 125

W

wart viruses (papilloma) 18, 66, 27, 97–100
water 17–23, 59, 61
weapons of mass destruction 128–30
West Nile virus 34–5, 49
white spot syndrome 18
World Health Organization (WHO) 38, 105 109–10, 125–6

X

xenotransplantation 130

Y

yellow fever 27, 122–4

Yuang Chan 94, 101

Z

zoonotic viruses 41–3,
119
zur Hausen, Herald 98

Viruses

Expand your collection of
VERY SHORT INTRODUCTIONS

1. Classics
2. Music
3. Buddhism
4. Literary Theory
5. Hinduism
6. Psychology
7. Islam
8. Politics
9. Theology
10. Archaeology
11. Judaism
12. Sociology
13. The Koran
14. The Bible
15. Social and Cultural Anthropology
16. History
17. Roman Britain
18. The Anglo-Saxon Age
19. Medieval Britain
20. The Tudors
21. Stuart Britain
22. Eighteenth-Century Britain
23. Nineteenth-Century Britain
24. Twentieth-Century Britain
25. Heidegger
26. Ancient Philosophy
27. Socrates
28. Marx
29. Logic
30. Descartes
31. Machiavelli
32. Aristotle
33. Hume
34. Nietzsche
35. Darwin
36. The European Union
37. Gandhi
38. Augustine
39. Intelligence
40. Jung
41. Buddha
42. Paul
43. Continental Philosophy
44. Galileo
45. Freud
46. Wittgenstein
47. Indian Philosophy
48. Rousseau
49. Hegel
50. Kant
51. Cosmology
52. Drugs
53. Russian Literature
54. The French Revolution
55. Philosophy
56. Barthes
57. Animal Rights
58. Kierkegaard
59. Russell
60. Shakespeare
61. Clausewitz
62. Schopenhauer
63. The Russian Revolution
64. Hobbes
65. World Music
66. Mathematics
67. Philosophy of Science

68. Cryptography
69. Quantum Theory
70. Spinoza
71. Choice Theory
72. Architecture
73. Poststructuralism
74. Postmodernism
75. Democracy
76. Empire
77. Fascism
78. Terrorism
79. Plato
80. Ethics
81. Emotion
82. Northern Ireland
83. Art Theory
84. Locke
85. Modern Ireland
86. Globalization
87. The Cold War
88. The History of Astronomy
89. Schizophrenia
90. The Earth
91. Engels
92. British Politics
93. Linguistics
94. The Celts
95. Ideology
96. Prehistory
97. Political Philosophy
98. Postcolonialism
99. Atheism
100. Evolution
101. Molecules
102. Art History
103. Presocratic Philosophy
104. The Elements
105. Dada and Surrealism
106. Egyptian Myth
107. Christian Art
108. Capitalism
109. Particle Physics
110. Free Will
111. Myth
112. Ancient Egypt
113. Hieroglyphs
114. Medical Ethics
115. Kafka
116. Anarchism
117. Ancient Warfare
118. Global Warming
119. Christianity
120. Modern Art
121. Consciousness
122. Foucault
123. The Spanish Civil War
124. The Marquis de Sade
125. Habermas
126. Socialism
127. Dreaming
128. Dinosaurs
129. Renaissance Art
130. Buddhist Ethics
131. Tragedy
132. Sikhism
133. The History of Time
134. Nationalism
135. The World Trade Organization
136. Design
137. The Vikings
138. Fossils
139. Journalism
140. The Crusades
141. Feminism
142. Human Evolution

143. The Dead Sea Scrolls
144. The Brain
145. Global Catastrophes
146. Contemporary Art
147. Philosophy of Law
148. The Renaissance
149. Anglicanism
150. The Roman Empire
151. Photography
152. Psychiatry
153. Existentialism
154. The First World War
155. Fundamentalism
156. Economics
157. International Migration
158. Newton
159. Chaos
160. African History
161. Racism
162. Kabbalah
163. Human Rights
164. International Relations
165. The American Presidency
166. The Great Depression and
     The New Deal
167. Classical Mythology
168. The New Testament as
     Literature
169. American Political Parties
     and Elections
170. Bestsellers
171. Geopolitics
172. Antisemitism
173. Game Theory
174. HIV/AIDS
175. Documentary Film
176. Modern China

177. The Quakers
178. German Literature
179. Nuclear Weapons
180. Law
181. The Old Testament
182. Galaxies
183. Mormonism
184. Religion in America
185. Geography
186. The Meaning of Life
187. Sexuality
188. Nelson Mandela
189. Science and Religion
190. Relativity
191. The History of Medicine
192. Citizenship
193. The History of Life
194. Memory
195. Autism
196. Statistics
197. Scotland
198. Catholicism
199. The United Nations
200. Free Speech
201. The Apocryphal Gospels
202. Modern Japan
203. Lincoln
204. Superconductivity
205. Nothing
206. Biography
207. The Soviet Union
208. Writing and Script
209. Communism
210. Fashion
211. Forensic Science
212. Puritanism
213. The Reformation

214. Thomas Aquinas
215. Deserts
216. The Norman Conquest
217. Biblical Archaeology
218. The Reagan Revolution
219. The Book of Mormon
220. Islamic History
221. Privacy
222. Neoliberalism
223. Progressivism
224. Epidemiology
225. Information
226. The Laws of Thermodynamics
227. Innovation
228. Witchcraft
229. The New Testament
230. French Literature
231. Film Music
232. Druids
233. German Philosophy
234. Advertising
235. Forensic Psychology
236. Modernism
237. Leadership
238. Christian Ethics
239. Tocqueville
240. Landscapes and Geomorphology
241. Spanish Literature
242. Diplomacy
243. North American Indians
244. The U.S. Congress
245. Romanticism
246. Utopianism
247. The Blues
248. Keynes
249. English Literature
250. Agnosticism
251. Aristocracy
252. Martin Luther
253. Michael Faraday
254. Planets
255. Pentecostalism
256. Humanism
257. Folk Music
258. Late Antiquity
259. Genius
260. Numbers
261. Muhammad
262. Beauty
263. Critical Theory
264. Organizations
265. Early Music
266. The Scientific Revolution
267. Cancer
268. Nuclear Power
269. Paganism
270. Risk
271. Science Fiction
272. Herodotus
273. Conscience
274. American Immigration
275. Jesus
276. Viruses